Manual of Embryo Culture in Human Assisted Reproduction

Cambridge Laboratory Manuals in Assisted Reproductive Technology

Titles in the series:

Manual of Embryo Culture in Human Assisted Reproduction

Edited by

Kersti Lundin
Sahlgrenska University Hospital

Aisling Ahlström
Livio Fertility Center

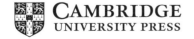

CAMBRIDGE
UNIVERSITY PRESS

University Printing House, Cambridge CB2 8BS, United Kingdom

One Liberty Plaza, 20th Floor, New York, NY 10006, USA

477 Williamstown Road, Port Melbourne, VIC 3207, Australia

314–321, 3rd Floor, Plot 3, Splendor Forum, Jasola District Centre, New Delhi – 110025, India

79 Anson Road, #06–04/06, Singapore 079906

Cambridge University Press is part of the University of Cambridge.

It furthers the University's mission by disseminating knowledge in the pursuit of education, learning, and research at the highest international levels of excellence.

www.cambridge.org
Information on this title: www.cambridge.org/9781108812610
DOI: 10.1017/9781108874014

First published 2021

Printed in the United Kingdom by TJ Books Ltd, Padstow Cornwall

A catalogue record for this publication is available from the British Library.

Library of Congress Cataloging-in-Publication Data
Names: Lundin, Kersti, editor. | Ahlström, Aisling, editor.
Title: Manual of embryo culture in human assisted reproduction / edited by Kersti Lundin, Aisling Ahlström.
Description: Cambridge, United Kingdom ; New York, NY : Cambridge University Press, 2020. | Includes bibliographical references and index. |
Identifiers: LCCN 2020042233 (print) | LCCN 2020042234 (ebook) | ISBN 9781108812610 (paperback) | ISBN 9781108874014 (epub)
Subjects: MESH: Embryo Culture Techniques | Fertilization in Vitro
Classification: LCC RG135 (print) | LCC RG135 (ebook) | NLM WQ 208 | DDC 618.1/780599–dc23
LC record available at https://lccn.loc.gov/2020042233
LC ebook record available at https://lccn.loc.gov/2020042234

ISBN 978-1-108-81261-0 Paperback

Contents

Contributors

Aisling Ahlström
Livio Fertility Center, Gothenburg, Sweden

Andrea Borini
9.baby Family and Fertility Center, Bologna, Italy

Giovanni Coticchio
9.baby Family and Fertility Center, Bologna, Italy

Carol Lynn Curchoe
CCRM Orange County, Newport Beach, CA, USA

John Dumoulin
Department of Obstetrics & Gynaecology, GROW
School for Oncology and Developmental Biology,
Maastricht University Medical Centre, the Netherlands

Thomas Freour
Service de médecine et biologie de la reproduction,
CHU de Nantes, Nantes, France & CRTI, Inserm,
Université de Nantes, Nantes, France

Julius Hreinsson
Minerva Fertility Clinic, Uppsala, Sweden

Hubert Joris
Research Department, Vitrolife, Gothenburg, Sweden

Borut Kovačič
Department of Reproductive Medicine and
Gynecological Endocrinology, University Medical
Centre Maribor, Slovenia

Kirstine Kirkegaard
Department of Obstetrics and Gynecology, Aarhus
University Hospital, Denmark

Kersti Lundin
Sahlgrenska University Hospital, Gothenburg,
Sweden

Thomas B. Pool
Fertility Center of San Antonio, San Antonio, Texas, USA

Michael L. Reed
The Fertility Center of New Mexico, Albuquerque,
New Mexico, USA

Ioannis Sfontouris
Division of Child Health, Obstetrics and
Gynaecology, University of Nottingham, UK
Hygeia IVF Athens, Greece

Roger G. Sturmey
Centre for Atherothrombosis and Metabolic Disease,
Hull York Medical School, University of Hull, UK

Arne Sunde
Department of Clinical and Molecular Medicine,
Norwegian University of Science and Technology,
Trondheim, Norway

Jason E. Swain
CCRM Fertility Network, Lone Tree, Colorado, USA

Kelly Tilleman
Department of Reproductive Medicine, Ghent
University Hospital, Belgium

Annelies Tolpe
Department of Reproductive Medicine, Ghent
University Hospital

Aafke van Montfoort
Department of Obstetrics & Gynaecology, GROW
School for Oncology and Developmental Biology,
Maastricht University Medical Centre, the
Netherlands

Paula Vergaro
Centre for Atherothrombosis and Metabolic Disease,
Hull York Medical School, University of Hull, UK

Carlotta Zacà
9.baby Family and Fertility Center, Bologna, Italy

Preface

Dear readers,

In a span of just a couple of decades, human reproduction has been revolutionized by the widespread use of assisted reproduction. Many couples and individuals who previously could not achieve pregnancy and live birth are now able to fulfill their wish for a family. In addition, it is possible to postpone and plan the time for reproduction through improved cryopreservation techniques for gametes and embryos.

Today, assisted reproduction techniques are established all over the world, having led to more than 9 million children being born, with an estimated more than 10 million embryos cryopreserved. It is important to remember that the success of these – now more or less standard – procedures have been accomplished by the dedicated work of a large number of scientists, embryologists and clinicians.

However, despite considerable experimental and clinical research, we still only have a partial understanding of what constitutes a "true" embryo environment. In vivo the oocyte travels from the ovary to the uterus through a landscape of changing physiological conditions. Much effort has been made to mimic this varying environment in in vitro culture but we still do not know whether, in the end, the embryos should be in utero for a better environment or maintained in vitro for a better selection. Research has been especially directed towards the composition of culture media, handling of the gametes and embryos, and the design of specialized incubators to create stable and controlled conditions regarding pH, temperature and osmolarity.

It is, however, clear that a successful IVF program is, to a large extent, due to the setup and performance of the laboratory and the laboratory staff. Culture of human embryos must be performed by trained and skilled staff, in laboratories conforming to strict guidelines, with specially adapted facilities and equipment. In addition, the IVF laboratory has increasingly developed into a highly technical facility, often requiring extra competencies and resources to maintain optimal performance.

The aim of this book is to cover all main aspects of culturing human embryos in vitro. For a start, a quality-controlled and well-functioning laboratory, including clean room standards and all equipment and consumables validated, controlled and traceable is mandatory. Standard operational procedures should be documented, adhered to and updated, and results monitored via benchmarking procedures. On a more basic level, we also need to determine more about the embryo itself: what are the nutritional needs and demands of an embryo and how should we accommodate the developing embryo to achieve the best outcome in terms of potential for implantation and live birth. However, we must never forget that the ultimate goal of assisted reproductive technology (ART) is the birth of a healthy child. It is, therefore, of the utmost importance to consider outcome not only as fertilization rates or implantation rates, but ultimately as the health of the offspring. We need to understand how we can use existing knowledge to improve embryo culture and development and minimize any impact on the health of future IVF children. Therefore, both current processes and future aspects including systems on the horizon that might be envisioned to enhance development of embryo culture and embryo handling must be continuously evaluated.

In this book the terms IVF, ART, and MAR (clinic/laboratory) are all used. According to the ICMART International Glossary, MAR (Medically Assisted Reproduction) is a broader term and refers to all treatments in assisted reproduction, including also, for example, hormonal stimulation and intrauterine insemination.

Considering all of the above, we are convinced that behind successful culture of embryos stands an educated and dedicated team working in well-equipped laboratories, supported by a structured and quality controlling management. We hope that this book will provide a comprehensive overview and a better understanding of how to provide and run such a system.

Many authors, all of them international experts in the field of reproductive science and medicine, have contributed to make this book possible. They have put a huge amount of time and work into providing excellent chapters, covering everything from the basics of human embryo culture to the most recent evidence. We are very grateful to all of you!

Kersti Lundin and Aisling Ahlström

Facilities for Embryo Culture

Julius Hreinsson

1.1 Background

Cell culture laboratories in general require facilities with very high standards of hygiene and air quality. Maintaining a Grade-A environment (ISO 4 or above) in these laboratories is usually necessary with respect to particle counts and airborne microbial colony forming units. This minimizes the risk of contamination and permits cell culture for prolonged periods of time.

In vitro fertilization (IVF) laboratories also require high standards of cleanliness, but in addition, special requirements add an element of increased complexity. For some aspects, compromises must be made between the most desirable standards and what is practically possible. This refers particularly to the necessity for close proximity to the operating room (OR) where oocyte retrievals and embryo transfers are performed, as well as other outpatient surgery such as testicular biopsies. The sensitive nature of the oocytes and embryos places certain restrictions on ventilation and disinfection. The relatively short culture period in IVF on the other hand allows for somewhat greater flexibility while other aspects place certain restrictions on attainment of Grade-A hygienic standards. This pertains particularly to temperature sensitivity and very low tolerance to toxic compounds, such as volatile organic compounds (VOCs) which, for example, places restrictions on the use of disinfectants such as alcohol (Morbeck 2015; Mortimer 2005).

The aim of this chapter is to describe the facilities and layout of an IVF laboratory and how the requisite quality and hygiene standards are met while conforming to applicable regulations.

The chapter will be organized according to the following sub-headings:

- General aspects of air quality
- Hygiene
- Layout of the laboratory and communication with the OR
- Laboratory storage
- Safety in the IVF laboratory
- Security for the IVF laboratory
- Gas and electrical power supply.

1.2 General Aspects of Air Quality in the IVF Laboratory

Human embryo culture is highly sensitive to airborne contaminants – particulate, microbial and organic – and requires high standards of air purity and quality. Therefore, it is necessary to place high demands on facilities for assisted reproductive technology (ART) laboratories to ensure optimal culture conditions. Some countries place strict demands through legislation and formal regulation whereas others work through guidelines. For example, since 2004 the European Union has had a directive in force to ensure high standards in ART laboratories (Hreinsson and Kovačič, 2019). There is also a wide consensus within the ART community that air quality in the IVF laboratory needs to meet certain criteria and that contaminants must be kept to a minimum (Esteves & Bento 2016; Mortimer et al., 2018). For a discussion on ISO classes of air quality vs. the GMP A–D classes, see Guns and Janssens (2019).

In general, the ART laboratory can be compared to an OR in terms of air quality and should be supplied with HEPA (high-efficiency particulate absorption) filtered air to achieve a comparable level of cleanliness. This requires at least ISO class 7 for air quality (see Table 1.1). It is recommended that the laboratory should be located in the middle of the facilities so that the laboratory does not lie adjacent to the outside walls or windows of the building. In essence, this means maintaining the "room within the

Table 1.1 Main criteria which must be met when designing and operating an IVF laboratory

Parameter	Details
Particulates	Maximum of 352,000 particles $\geq$0.5 μm
Airborne microorganisms	Maximum of 10 colony forming units per m^3 Maximum of 5 colony forming units per 90 mm settle plate
VOCs	<60 ppb
Air changes	15–20 per hour
Overpressure	Minimum of +30 Pa
Temperature	22–24°C
Humidity	40–50%
Air filtration	HEPA
Carbon and potassium permanganate filtration	Built into the HVAC system

For further details, see Mortimer et al. (2018).

room" principle, facilitating the maintenance of air purity and decreasing the risk for contamination.

It is well established that VOCs can have a detrimental effect on human embryo culture (Esteves & Bento, 2016). Materials used when building the laboratory, including flooring and wall covering as well as furniture and equipment, should have low off-gassing rates, and the entire laboratory in new or renovated facilities should be allowed a burn-off period of several weeks before being taken into use.

The HVAC system (heating, ventilation and air conditioning) is highly important and usually the laboratory and OR run on a separate, isolated system. Typically the HVAC system is installed during construction since most buildings do not have sufficient capacity in the regular systems. By including carbon and potassium permanganate filters in the ventilation system, toxic VOCs can be absorbed and removed from the air flowing into the laboratory. All filters in the HVAC system must be monitored and maintained regularly with replacements scheduled as necessary. To reduce the burden on these filters, the location of the air intake for the HVAC system must also be considered. Usually these are placed on the top of the building to avoid car exhaust and other contaminants which can be a problem in large cities. In hospitals, helicopter platforms on the roof of the building may also create complications and need to be taken into consideration.

The number of air changes in a room of ISO class 7 should be 60–150 per hour. However, IVF laboratories usually aim at 15–20 air changes per hour with only part of the air flow coming directly from the air intake and the rest being recirculated. This is because too high air flow rates may impact temperature stability of heating zones and in culture dishes and also increase evaporation rates from culture droplets during culture media preparation. Here, a balance must be found between air quality and maintaining general physical parameters within acceptable ranges. Laminar flow hoods are to be used for preparation of the dishes to counteract this potential problem.

Maintaining humidity levels between 40% and 50% in the laboratory is optimal since lower levels will increase microdroplet evaporation whereas higher levels may induce formation of mold. There is also the issue of maintaining a healthy environment for staff. The same applies to temperature in the laboratory which should be kept at a level ensuring a comfortable environment. A high room temperature is not optimal for incubators which are designed to run at a temperature differential of approximately 13–15°C above ambient surroundings.

It is standard for all clean rooms to have a positive pressure differential from the laboratory to their surroundings. This will reduce the risk of contaminants entering the laboratory from the outside. This pertains to general air contaminants as above but is also relevant to the OR since the disinfectants and cleaning agents necessary for optimal patient care must not carry over into the laboratory. Each laboratory needs to be able to perform tests to determine particle counts, microbial contamination, and VOCs in the air in the facilities.

Typically, an ART clinic operates as an outpatient clinic with minor surgery under local anesthesia only, the great majority of patients being ambulatory. Although emergency provisions and access for persons with disabilities should be possible in the facilities, this is usually feasible in office buildings as well. If general anesthesia and more invasive surgery are to be performed in the facilities, this places additional demands on patient monitoring, emergency access and around the clock availability. When planning general anesthesia and more invasive surgery, separate demands must be met. This chapter does not address the issues raised in these cases

1.3 Hygiene

When operating a clean laboratory with adequate ventilation and filtration, it becomes clear that the staff is a major source of particle contamination in the IVF laboratory. Therefore the use of non-shedding clothing and hair covers is mandatory in the IVF laboratory. Gloves are used for personal protection when working with body fluids, such as sperm samples or follicle aspirates. In addition, the use of masks is recommended in certain instances, such as when performing embryo biopsy and tubing for preimplantation genetic testing. Hand hygiene must be observed at all times since use of gloves is often considered inconvenient and possibly risky when working with fine manipulation, as in the IVF laboratory setting. Rings, wrist watches, and jewelry should not be worn in the OR or in the laboratory, as is the general hospital standard. In addition to soap and water, hand disinfectants which do not emit VOCs should be used.

Use of alcohol for disinfection in the laboratory is normally discouraged because of the potential toxic effects associated with it. Although using alcohol on work surfaces in a well-ventilated laboratory after all cell culture work has been performed may be in order, especially when using incubators with closed gas circulation, it is generally avoided. Instead quaternary ammonium compounds which do not emit VOCs can be used, or hydrogen peroxide solutions which do not leave a residue after use. Each laboratory needs to verify and validate the cleaning methods used as well as establishing general hygienic

standards, finding a balance between maintaining good hygiene and avoiding infections while minimizing any potential toxic effects to the gametes and embryos.

All work areas must be thoroughly cleaned both in terms of pathogens but also to avoid DNA-contamination in embryology laboratories performing preimplantation genetic testing. Supplies in cardboard boxes must never enter the laboratory (see 1.5 Laboratory Storage). Administrative work should be minimized in the laboratory and OR covers for computers should be considered.

To facilitate cleaning of the rooms, sealed mats with rounded corners should be used for the floor and the ceiling should be sealed with rounded corners as well. Lights should be built into the ceiling. Proper floor material, such as metal sheets, should be used where liquid nitrogen is handled. If windows are exposed to direct sunlight, dark shades need to be applied.

The laboratory and OR should be tested for airborne microorganisms using sedimentation plates or specialized measuring devices to evaluate the standard of the air quality in this respect.

The issue of lighting in the IVF-laboratory often comes up. As a general rule, low intensity lighting is recommended while maintaining a safe and secure working environment is paramount. When considering light sources in the IVF-laboratory, it is useful to consider that oocytes and embryos are kept in incubators most of the time and are not exposed to ambient light. The majority of light exposure to the ovum and embryo occurs during microscopic examination and micromanipulation. The light sources in the microscopes are typically halogen light bulbs from 30 watts up to 100 watts and the operator can minimize this exposure by using the lowest possible intensity required to perform the work (Ottosen et al., 2007). Use of colored light filters can be considered as well.

Ambient light should be reduced and direct sunlight cannot be allowed in the IVF laboratory.

1.4 Layout of the Laboratory

As mentioned previously, there are many advantages if the laboratory is designed as a "room within the room," i.e., having a corridor or other rooms between the laboratory and the outside walls. The laboratory should also not open up directly to the surrounding clinic but should be entered through an air lock or vestibule used for hand washing, change of footwear, donning masks, and hair covers etc. A changing room for staff should be located in the vicinity of the laboratory and laboratory coats should be available for guests. As a rule, sinks for hand washing and for cleaning instruments should not be located within the clean room laboratory. These can be placed in the vestibule.

The embryology laboratory should be located next to the OR to facilitate safe and swift transfer of oocytes and embryos. Although the OR should be accessible from the laboratory by a door, transfer of follicular aspirates and embryo transfer catheters, should preferentially be achieved through a window or hatch, which can be closed between operations. By locating the workstation by the window on the laboratory side, the embryologist and physician can work close to each other and tubes with follicular aspirates or embryo transfer catheters can easily and quickly be transferred between the OR and laboratory. This minimizes staffing and also maximizes patient integrity during the procedure while improving quality and ease of operations.

Each workstation in the laboratory should allow for a computer station to facilitate registration in the Electronic Medical Records system (EMR) and an electronic witnessing system should also be incorporated in the work station to minimize risk for identification errors (see details in Chapter 7).

It is often considered practical to place the incubators in the center of the laboratory with the gas lines coming from the ceiling. Separate work stations can then be located around the periphery of the laboratory allowing for easy access to the long-term culture incubators. The laboratory should be planned in such a way that the distance from any given working station to the long-term culture incubator is as short as possible to minimize walking with dishes containing oocytes or embryos.

Each work station in the laboratory should be equipped with a laminar flow hood and a zoom stereo microscope. The specifications for these microscopes may vary, as typically low magnification is needed for oocyte retrieval and embryo transfer whereas higher magnification may be required for more advanced manipulation and evaluation. All embryo evaluation is performed at the inverted microscope (or through time lapse monitoring) at $200\times$ magnification (ESHRE Guideline Group et al., 2016). Also the work stations should be separated with respect to working on warm vs. room temperature surfaces. For example it is preferable that vitrification work stations are located closer to liquid nitrogen supply than the intracytoplasmic sperm injection (ICSI) or embryo biopsy workstations.

While vitrification and cryopreservation are performed in the embryology and andrology laboratories, long-term storage of samples may be better achieved in a separate facility. This becomes particularly pertinent if a large number of samples are stored, as in larger laboratories with gamete banks or those performing fertility preservation banking for oncology patients. Here, ease of access should be considered for filling the nitrogen supply tanks because of the large volumes of liquid nitrogen required. Storing numerous large dewars in the IVF laboratory itself is not recommended.

The andrology laboratory should be located in the vicinity of the embryology laboratory. The general principles as specified above also apply there. It is useful to have direct access between embryology and andrology and in smaller facilities an "andrology corner" can be a part of the embryology laboratory. The work stations in andrology are by necessity different with Class II flow hoods being preferable and with a small centrifuge included in the hood. It is highly recommended to plan andrology and the number of work stations in such a way that one sample can be processed at a time in a dedicated flow hood and with a dedicated andrologist while using electronic witnessing systems.

1.5 Laboratory Storage

Every IVF laboratory requires a dedicated storage area for supplies. In order to maintain a high standard, supplies must be unpacked outside the laboratory itself and cartons must not be brought into the IVF laboratory. Ideally, two storage areas should be used – the first for supplies coming in and the second for batches which have been tested and/or approved for use. This setup allows for optimal supply management ensuring that the first-come-first-use principle is adhered to and also that only approved materials are in use in the laboratory.

1.6 Safety in the IVF Laboratory

The IVF laboratory uses liquid nitrogen for cryopreservation and cryostorage in vacuum isolated dewars. In many cases large volumes of liquid nitrogen are handled by the laboratory, often hundreds of liters. This raises two safety issues.

Firstly, liquid nitrogen expands 696 times when it evaporates and atmospheric oxygen may be depleted if the facilities are not well ventilated. Large volumes of nitrogen gas may be emitted in cases of tank failure. Therefore all facilities with nitrogen storage must be equipped with an oxygen depletion alarm for safety. The alarm should have both visual and audible signals and should be sent through the general alarm channels (see Section 1.7 Security in the IVF Laboratory). In large storage facilities, for safety, access is permitted only for at least two persons simultaneously.

Secondly, because of the extremely low temperature of the liquid ($-196°C$), working with liquid nitrogen confers certain risks. Thermoisolated gloves, goggles, and isolation aprons as well as shoes which completely cover the operators feet should be available and used.

Most IVF laboratories are from time to time required to handle samples from patients with known viral infections. Personal protection in the form of gloves and visor should be considered and processing of these samples should be performed separately from other samples. At least, these samples should be separated in time from other samples and through cleaning performed afterwards. Good laboratory practice includes using gloves when processing sperm samples, identifying oocytes from follicle fluid and during embryo transfer.

It is advisable to consider ergonomics when planning the IVF laboratory. Work stations with adjustable height allow for varying working positions and also for adapting to optimal working positions for each individual. Ergonomically adjustable microscopes and other equipment allow for long-term working in the IVF laboratory while maintaining good posture and health (Hreinsson & Borg, 2019).

1.7 Security in the IVF Laboratory

All areas where cells and tissues are handled and/or stored need to maintain strict access control. This is easy to achieve using modern systems where access is coupled with an individual's identification card. This affords the added advantage of complete traceability of who has entered the laboratory and when. All visitors must sign confidentiality agreements and must be accompanied by a designated supervisor for the visit. Facilities should be equipped with an intruder alarm after hours.

IVF culture and cryostorage is maintained around the clock, whereas clinical procedures are usually performed during daytime. Therefore it is essential that all critical equipment is linked to an external alarm system with separate monitoring of critical parameters such as temperature and gas levels. This includes incubators, nitrogen tanks, refrigerators, gas manifolds, and others. Calibration of sensors is performed according to international standards. Staff may take turns carrying a portable alarm or a single person may take responsibility of monitoring alarms. Alarms must be monitored and tested regularly and trends in critical parameters, such as temperature, should be analyzed. Laboratories with large volumes of samples in cryostorage do well to have reserve tanks in case of tank failure as such an event only allows for only a few hours response time before samples are at risk of being compromised (Pomeroy & Marcon, 2018). Typically the alarm systems monitor temperature, both in incubators and also in the nitrogen dewars. However, a weight-based monitoring system may also have advantages and can be considered (Michaelson et al., 2019).

The issue of gas phase vs. liquid phase storage at nitrogen temperatures often comes up. Typically samples of larger volume, such as sperm samples, are stored in the gas phase as this is considered safer regarding possible contamination. Smaller volume samples, such as vitrified oocytes and embryos, can be stored in the gas phase of liquid nitrogen and this is the rule during transport. However, many embryologists are concerned that this will increase risk of premature warming during handling so long-term liquid nitrogen storage is often recommended for these samples.

1.8 Gas and Electrical Power

The gas manifold and nitrogen supply are usually located outside the IVF laboratory and on the ground floor to allow for cleanliness as well as to ensure easy access and delivery.

The IVF laboratory typically requires three types of gas which should be supplied through stainless steel tubing, not copper. These are CO_2, N_2 and a gas mixture for culture (6% CO_2, 5% O_2 and 89% N_2, for example). The gas manifold should be included in the alarm system and located outside of the laboratory itself. The gas lines do not require high pressure but if the laboratory is located several levels above the ground floor, this must of course be taken into consideration. Redundancy and automatic switching to full gas tanks is necessary.

In addition to the laboratory gas supply, the OR requires medical gases, such as oxygen.

Any IVF laboratory will experience power outages from time to time. Therefore it is important that critical equipment is connected to an uninterrupted power supply such as a UPS battery backup supply. A local generator may be in place for long-term power shortages, but the battery backup must be in place for uninterrupted power. It should be considered that some equipment in the IVF laboratory, such as flow hoods, are sensitive to power surges and may be negatively affected by power outages even though they are not part of the culture system itself.

1.9 Conclusions

Facilities for the IVF laboratory and adjacent ORs need to be carefully planned and designed to allow for safe and efficient workflow. One of the main areas of focus is ensuring high standards of air quality to allow for a safe culture environment. Provisions for technical, safety and security measures for continuous monitoring, culture, and storage of gametes and embryos need to be made and upheld in all ART facilities.

References

ESHRE Guideline Group on Good Practice in IVF Labs, De los Santos MJ, Apter S, et al. Revised guidelines for good practice in IVF laboratories (2015). *Hum Reprod.* 2016;31:685–686.

Esteves SC, Bento FC. Air quality control in the ART laboratory is a major determinant of IVF success. *Asian J Androl.* 2016;18:596–599.

Guns J, Janssens R. Air quality management. In: Nagy Z, Varghese A, Agarwal A, eds. *In Vitro Fertilization: A Textbook of Current and Emerging Methods and Devices.* 2nd edn. Cham: Springer; 2019.

Hreinsson J, Borg K. Risk and safety in the IVF Clinic. In: Nagy Z, Varghese A, Agarwal A, eds. *In Vitro Fertilization: A Textbook of Current and Emerging Methods and Devices.* 2nd edn. Cham: Springer; 2019.

Hreinsson J, Kovačič B. Regulation, licensing, and accreditation of the ART laboratory in Europe. In: Nagy Z, Varghese A, Agarwal A, eds. *In Vitro Fertilization: A Textbook of Current and Emerging Methods and Devices.* 2nd edn. Cham: Springer; 2019.

Michaelson ZP, Bondalapati ST, Amrane S, et al. Early detection of cryostorage tank failure using a weight-based monitoring system. *J Assist Reprod Genet.* 2019;36:655–660.

Morbeck DE. Air quality in the assisted reproduction laboratory: a mini-review. *J Assist Reprod Genet.* 2015;32:1019–1024.

Mortimer D. A critical assessment of the impact of the European Union Tissues and Cells Directive (2004) on laboratory practices in assisted conception. *Reprod Biomed Online.* 2005;11:162–176.

Mortimer D, Cohen J, Mortimer ST, et al. Cairo consensus on the IVF laboratory environment and air quality: report of an expert meeting. *Reprod Biomed Online.* 2018;36:658–674.

Ottosen LD, Hindkjaer J, Ingerslev J. Light exposure of the ovum and preimplantation embryo during ART procedures. *J Assist Reprod Genet.* 2007;24(2-3):99–103.

Pomeroy KO, Marcon M. Reproductive tissue storage: Quality control and management/inventory software. *Semin Reprod Med.* 2018;36:280–288.

Chapter 2

Incubators for Embryo Culture

Borut Kovačič

2.1 Introduction

Incubators represent the most important piece of equipment in an in vitro fertilization (IVF) laboratory since embryos spend the largest part of their in vitro development within an incubator's atmosphere. Incubators, together with embryo culture media, are intended to directly and indirectly provide stable physicochemical conditions that best mimic the natural environment in the female reproductive tract. The stability of these conditions significantly influences the success of the IVF program. Modern incubators can be very sophisticated devices that can be upgraded with integrated micro cameras and linked to computer programs. Although the incubator's technical details may sometimes be difficult to understand, it is important for clinical embryologists to know how to control incubator operation and properly maintain stable physical and hygienic conditions.

When considering investment in IVF laboratory equipment, it makes sense to first think about incubators. The decision about which type of incubator would best meet the requirements of the laboratory is not easy because of the wide range of different types of incubators. This chapter describes the characteristics of the various types of incubators and the related physical and chemical factors affecting embryo development.

2.2 Incubator Types

During the early period of cell culture development, and even later with the first human embryos being cultured in vitro, a glass jar (desiccator) placed into a heating chamber controlled by a thermostat was used as an incubator. Distilled water was poured into the lower part of the jar to ensure a sufficiently high relative humidity in the space. This system was the first "air-jacket" CO_2 incubator, and the first IVF baby was conceived with the help of this type of incubator.[1]

During the 1960s, the first commercial CO_2 incubators were developed by New Brunswick Scientific (New Jersey, USA). In 1984, Shel Lab (Cornelius, USA) introduced the general purpose incubator, which had a warm air jacket, heated door, and five integrated heating elements to maintain a uniform temperature, with no hot spots. Gas concentrations were monitored by thermocouple sensors, which were very sensitive to temperature and humidity. Different companies launched many similar types of incubators, almost all with installed fans to enable equal physical conditions in all parts of the chamber.

At the beginning of the 2000s, a new line of CO_2 incubators appeared on the market, featuring a direct-heat and fanless design. These incubators were lighter than water-jacketed incubators and had advanced infrared (IR) CO_2 sensors, working without sensitivity to other physical parameters. The incubator's interior became a seamless, deep-drawn inner stainless steel chamber. Such simplification of the interior facilitated easier cleaning and prevented contamination. The humidification system was also simplified and water condensation was prevented. They also contained their own LCD screens and on-board diagnostics.

Benchtop incubators were developed during the 1990s. Benchtop models modified for IVF (e.g., FIV series from Carteau, Bagnolet, France) had integrated microplates and a humidification system. This innovation offered optimal temperature uniformity and stability in 4-well culture dishes. The incubators had a simple construction in which multiple incubation chambers were stacked.

In the last decade, the evolution of embryonic culture incubators has been marked by the idea of placing a time-lapse (TL) microcamera inside a classic incubator (Primovision, Vitrolife, Göteborg, Sweden), enabling the continuous monitoring of embryo development. Linking TL cameras to appropriate software has opened up a new dimension in clinical embryology, being able to document the embryo continuously throughout the time of culture (more details on time-lapse in Chapter 10). One of the biggest advantages TL incubators provide is uninterrupted embryo culture as daily embryo scoring can be performed without removing the culture dish from the incubator.

2.2.1 Selection of Incubators

The development of incubators in recent years has made incredible progress. IVF laboratories can hardly adapt to such rapid development of technology, as it is resource demanding to replace all old incubators with new ones overnight. Therefore, in today's IVF laboratories, it is possible to find all types of incubators (Figures 2.1 and 2.2) with different technical characteristics (Table 2.1).

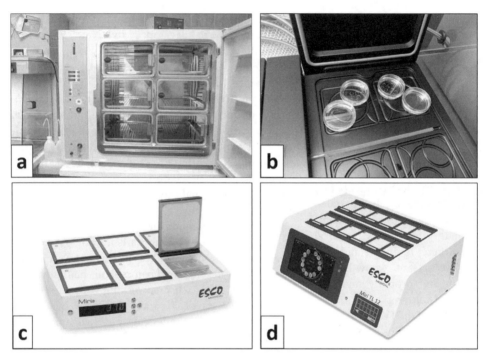

Figure 2.1 Incubators for overnight or longer embryo culture: **a.** large-box incubator; **b.** benchtop incubator; **c.** benchtop multi-room incubator; **d.** time-lapse incubator. For color version of this figure. Please refer color plate section.

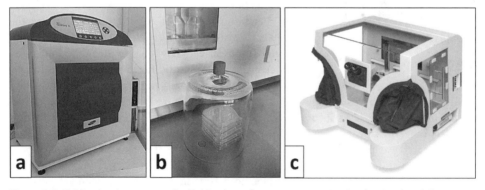

Figure 2.2 Holding incubators: **a.** smaller box incubator for sperm preparation; **b.** glass jar placed above an opening in the surface of the laminar flow through which CO_2 is introduced; **c.** closed workstation with controlled incubation atmosphere and integrated microscope. For color version of this figure. Please refer color plate section.

Table 2.1 Types of incubators for human IVF and their technical characteristics

Type	Technical properties and options	
Classic side-door incubators for overnight or longer culture: • Large-box incubators • Smaller box incubators	- Water jacket - Single door - Heated doors - Stainless steel chamber and shelves - Active humidification - Thermocouple CO_2 sensors - Galvanic O_2 sensors - Passively circulated air - Single gas port - CO_2 or gas mixture - Gas mixing system - O_2 control - Air filtration - Air sterilization by UV - Chamber heat sterilization - Chamber disinfection - Display line diagram option - Memorizing values - On-board diagnostics - RS232 port - Alarm	- Air jacket - Multiple doors - Non-heated doors - Cooper chamber and shelves - Passive humidification - Infrared CO_2 sensors - Zirconium O_2 sensors - Fan circulated air - Double gas ports - CO_2 and N_2 - No gas mixing system - No O_2 control - No air filtration - No UV - No heat sterilization - No disinfection - No line diagram options - No display of history - No diagnostics - No RS232 port - No alarm
Multichamber incubators for overnight or longer culture: • Drawer incubators • Benchtop incubators • Time-lapse benchtop incubators	- Individual chambers - Heated microplates adjusted to specific petri dish brands - General sensor for temperature and heating elements for all compartments - Mixed gas connection; single gas port - Gas filtration - Shared provision of mixed gas into all compartments through one gas line - Dry culture system - Built-in pH measuring system - Display line diagram - Memorizing values - On-board diagnostics - RS232 port - Alarm - For further technical characteristics and options for TL benchtop incubators, see ESHRE recommendation paper.[2]	- Shared chambers - Non-adjusted microplates to specific Petri dish brands - Individual sensor for temperature and heating elements for each compartment - Integrated gas mixer; separated gas ports - No gas filtration - Provision of mixed gas into each compartment through separated gas lines - Humid culture system - No pH measuring system - No line diagram option - No history - No diagnostics - No RS232 port - No alarm
Holding and/or working incubators for keeping culture media, gametes, embryos in a CO_2 culture atmosphere for a short period during handling with oocytes and embryos	Smaller box incubators, located near or within laminar flow cabinets. Glass jars or metal lids for covering petri dishes, with gas tubing connection or positioned on the gas exit opening on the laminar flow hood heating plate.	

Table 2.1 (*cont.*)

Type	Technical properties and options
• Smaller box working incubators • Lid incubators • Combined incubator–workstation	Hermetically closed combined incubator–workstation with controlled temperature and gases and with integrated microscope.
Other types • Sealed bag incubators • In vivo incubators • Microfluidic incubators	Sealed plastic bags, filled with gas mixture and sunk into a warm water bath (more appropriate for veterinary IVF). In vivo embryo culture or intravaginal embryo culture in closed tubes, permeable for gases from vagina. Closed device connected to the tubing system that enables constant circulation of culture medium around embryos.

Among the available incubators in the laboratory, it is necessary to identify those that will be used for overnight or extended culture of embryos to restrict the frequency of opening, and those that will serve as holding or working incubators. Holding and working incubators are dedicated to the preincubation of culture media and for short-term incubation, e.g., during sperm preparation, oocyte pick-up, fertilization, and cryopreservation.

While using large incubators, it is recommended that petri dishes with biological material from no more than one patient/couple should be kept on each shelf (or material from four to six patients in each incubator). With benchtop incubators, the recommendation is that only one patient's gametes/embryos should be cultured per incubator compartment.[3] In this way, the physical perturbation of the culture environment and the risk of a sample mix-up are reduced to a minimum. Time-lapse incubators and single-step media can enable uninterrupted embryo culture to the blastocyst stage. In addition, continuous monitoring of the morphodynamics of embryonic development and identification of embryo cleavage irregularities are possible, without any opening of the chamber.[2] Despite the remarkable advances in incubator technology, it is still difficult to claim that certain types provide better clinical results. Several studies have been conducted to compare the laboratory and clinical performance indicators after using large-box and small benchtop incubators for human gamete and embryo culture.[4] Some differences in embryo development have been observed between two types of incubators in a few studies.[5,6] However,

critical analysis identified limitations in the study design and when interpreting results with lack of consideration for many confounding variables that make it impossible to identify the effect of the incubator alone (see also Chapter 10). Most other trials demonstrate some differences in the culture parameters, but they could not confirm differences in any endpoint between incubators.[7–9] Nevertheless, from all comparisons made between different types of incubators, it is apparent that smaller compartments provide more rapid recovery of the temperature and gas concentration. This definitively results in less stress for oocytes and embryos, presumably resulting in improved embryo quality, which is also a goal of clinical embryology (see also Chapter 8).

Even though the embryo culture conditions have improved with new incubator types, many ART techniques still require manipulation of oocytes or embryos outside incubators (such as oocyte pick-ups, oocyte denudation, cryopreservation, ICSI, embryo biopsy, artificial blastocoel collapsing). Due to variations in physicochemical parameters during the performance of these techniques, they represent the most sensitive part of the IVF procedure and cause the most stress to oocytes and embryos. Some laboratories avoid this by using smaller working, non-culture box or lid incubators integrated into laminar flow benches. Glass or metal funnels, connected to a mixed gas source (Figure 2.2b), are also practical for maintaining culture conditions by using them to cover dishes during procedures. Even more stable conditions during oocyte and embryo manipulations can be achieved in a closed workstation with regulated temperature and in some cases also regulated gas concentration (Figure 2c). The performance of key IVF procedures, as those mentioned above, in a controlled atmosphere of closed laminar flow hoods can significantly improve clinical results.[10]

2.3 Installation

Before a new incubator is used for embryo culture, it must be properly cleaned and properly validated (Figure 2.3). It is recommended that authorized technical staff connect the new incubator to the electrical outlet and to the gas connections and set-up desired values in the menu. During the test run it is also advisable to keep the incubator out of the IVF laboratory, as the installation process, parameter setting, and incubator calibration / validation are expected to be a time-consuming process that may interfere with routine IVF work. In the laboratory, the incubator should be located near the laminar flow hood and connected to a permanent power source (uninterrupted power source, i.e., battery or generator).

Gas bottles should be installed outside the laboratory and automatically connect to a second gas bottle as soon as the first gas bottle is empty. Gas cylinders should be of the appropriate gas pressure scale to prevent too low or too high pressure on the incubator's gas connections. The gases exist in various purity grades. Although installing HEPA/VOC filters on gas tubing is recommended, the source of gases used for human embryo culture should also be of the highest purity (medical gases). Bottles containing a single gas enable a more constant gas supply in comparison with bottles with a gas mixture, but they require an integrated gas mixing system. When gases of desired concentrations are premixed, they can disperse differently in the bottle over time according to their specific weight and other physical properties. In both cases, the permanent independent control of gases in the incubation chamber is required to achieve a well-controlled and constant incubation atmosphere.

2.4 Cleaning and Preventing Contamination

Cleanliness is necessary to prevent contamination and microbial growth in incubators. Air movement in the laboratory can carry particles and microorganisms.

Even when all measures for preventing contamination are taken properly, the air will always contain some microorganisms and dust particles, most of which originates from the normal flora on the skin or from material brought in to the laboratory. This means that contaminants can enter the incubator each time the door is opened. The incubators should be positioned away from the floor. No items should be stored on top of the incubators because this prevents proper cleaning, and dust and dirt can be swept inside the chamber during door opening.

Cleaning agents recommended by the manufacturer are advisable for the initial and routine cleaning. For the initial cleaning of the interior, a mild non-perfumed detergent may be used, which needs to be well rinsed off the surface. As an alternative, hydrogen peroxide can be used to remove the proteins if the culture media have been spilled. Seventy percent alcohol was used for decontamination during routine maintenance in the past. Later, the alcohol was replaced by non-volatile disinfectants (e.g., Barricidal, Fertisafe). The more complex the incubator's interior, the more difficult it is to clean. In the case of conventional big volume incubators, shelves and the inner frame must be removed during cleaning and each part cleaned separately. When hot sterilization is performed, attention must be paid to the gas sensors. In some types of incubators, the sensors must be removed before sterilization. However, new types of big incubators already have heat-insensitive sensors.

The cleaning of benchtop incubators is much simpler; however, manufacturer's instructions must be followed. Internal heating plates can be easily wiped with alcohol, and in some benchtop incubators, they may even be removed and immersed in a disinfectant. Greater attention should be paid to water tubing systems that serve to supply moisture in some types of wet-culture incubators as these can be a source of contamination. Regular replacement of HEPA / VOC filters at the gas inlet is also part of the regular provision of hygienic standards.

The cleaning interval depends on the load of work in the laboratory as well as the frequency of usage. Each laboratory determines its own cleaning schedule. Incubators intended for sperm incubation require more frequent cleaning and are a more critical group of appliances as regards contamination compared to embryo culture incubators. Such incubators should have the option of hot sterilization.

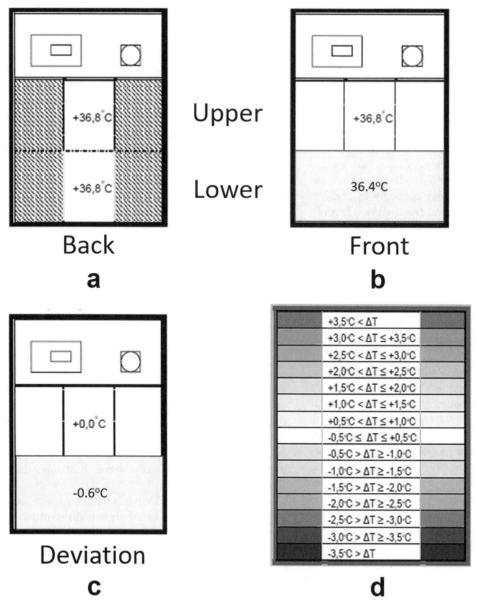

Figure 2.3 Incubator temperature validation report: **a.** measured temperature deep inside the chamber; **b.** measured temperature in the chamber near the door; **c.** deviation from the set temperature shown by the specific color of the deviation scale; **d.** color scale of temperature deviations from set point. For color version of this figure. Please refer color plate section.

After the completion of cleaning or sterilization, the proper functioning regarding temperature, gas levels, and pH of the incubators and their sensors must be checked, and the time for chamber ventilation must be enabled before they can be put back into use.

2.5 Functioning

The main function of an incubator is to regulate certain physical and, indirectly, chemical parameters that provide optimal conditions for an optimal embryo culture. The key physical parameters maintained by incubators are temperature and CO_2 concentration. The latter has an important indirect role in maintaining the physiological pH of the culture media. Physiological O_2 concentration, which is substantially below atmospheric O_2 levels, and relative humidity, which maintains a stable osmolality of the media, are also optional parameters. The optional parameters, reduced O_2 concentration and relative humidity, and their effect on embryonal development in incubators, have been the subject of numerous studies in the fields of clinical embryology in the past decade. No less important is the fact that the incubator can also be used to maintain clean air and, using an appropriate filter system, maintain a dust-free and VOC-free atmosphere.[11] Last but not least, among the most important functions of incubators is the requirement to recover the factors listed above as soon as possible after each time the incubator is opened.

2.5.1 Gas Systems

Regulation of gas concentrations in the incubator's atmosphere is crucial. The incubator types are chosen depending on what kind of atmosphere will be used for the embryo culture: atmospheric or reduced O_2. Incubators installed with a gas mixing system use a single gas connection (CO_2 inlet) and a CO_2 sensor to enable regulation of gas input. Incubators with regulated CO_2 and O_2 have separate CO_2 and O_2 sensors and separate gas inlets for CO_2 and N_2. The CO_2 sensors should be independent from other physical factors as much as possible. In contrast with thermal resistant CO_2 sensors, the infrared CO_2 sensors detect how much CO_2 is in the atmosphere by measuring how much 4.3 μm light passes through it. The amount of light detected is not dependent on other factors, such as humidity or temperature.[12]

Some incubators are able to achieve the physiological concentration of gases in the absence of CO_2 and O_2 sensors. They are connected to a bottle containing the desired gas mixture.

Both gas consumption and equilibration time vary significantly after opening large (150–200 l) or benchtop (0.3–0.5 l) incubators.

The pressure of the atmospheric air depends upon the altitude at which these objects are situated. The higher the altitude, the lower the pressure. If the altitude is not taken into account, the incubation atmosphere with a setting value of 5% O_2 or even lower can caused anoxic conditions for embryos. Modern incubators usually contain a menu which asks for the altitude before the setting points for other gas parameters are defined. In laboratories positioned at higher altitudes, the gas mixture can be an option, particularly if incubators do not have the menu system considering the altitude.

2.5.2 Incubation Environment

2.5.2.1 Carbon Dioxide

Regulation of the CO_2 concentration is the most important role of an incubator, since the CO_2 regulates the pH of the culture media. The pH is the result of the CO_2 concentration and the amount of bicarbonate in the culture medium. The CO_2 molecules are dissolved in the culture medium and produce carbonic acid that tends to reach equilibrium with dissolved bicarbonate: the higher the CO_2 concentration in the incubation atmosphere, the lower the pH of the medium.[13]

Complex measurements of media, by using specific pH measuring systems, are required for accurate information about their pH, as it is difficult to quantify. In a bicarbonate buffered medium, the pH starts to increase rapidly when the sample is exposed to the air. Stabilization of the correct media pH to maintain homeostasis is crucial for the minimization of intracellular stress and optimization of embryo development.

2.5.2.2 Oxygen

In the oviducts of rabbits, hamsters, and Rhesus monkeys, the O_2 concentration (partial pressure) has been shown to vary between 5% and 8.7% (38–66 mm Hg),[14] while in the uterine cavity it dropped to 3% to 5% (22–38 mm Hg) in rodents and to less than 2% (15 mmHg) in bovines, Rhesus monkeys, and humans.[15]

In the early period of human IVF, for almost the whole first decade, ART laboratories tried to mimic physiologic O_2 conditions and were equipped with CO_2 incubators, which provided a reduced (5%) O_2 atmosphere.[16–18] However, the relatively high pregnancy rate achieved by the transfer of embryos which have been successfully developed in atmospheric (20%) O_2 concentrations slowly led to the abandoning of low-O_2 equipment and to a decrease in costs related to the supply of a high amount of nitrogen.

The birth of more than 5 million children conceived in high O_2 culture conditions demonstrated that human embryos can tolerate up to atmospheric O_2 concentration.

Many physiological studies on mammalian embryos in vitro from the last 30 years clearly showed that atmospheric O_2 concentration could significantly change some physiological pathways in embryonic cells and negatively affect the gene expression, epigenetics, metabolism, and amino acid and carbohydrate turnover, and consequently the development of embryos to the blastocyst stage.[19] Furthermore, clinical studies showed a reduced O_2 concentration in the incubation atmosphere to be beneficial when used throughout the entire culture period to the blastocyst stage.[20]

Due to all of these reasons, a reduced O_2 concentration for human embryo culture is strongly recommended[21] and most manufacturers have already integrated the O_2 regulation in all of their CO_2 incubators for IVF use.

2.5.2.3 Temperature

Early on, the temperature of 37°C was accepted as the best temperature for all aspects of human in vitro procedures.[22]) Studies on the determination of the physiological values of temperature for gametes and embryos showed that the temperature in the upper fallopian tubes is lower and suggested that the incubator temperature should also be set lower to fully ensure physiological conditions.[23]) (See more in Chapter 8).

Heating in box-type incubators is provided by heaters in the outer jacket of the incubator. This may be a water- or air-jacket, but the latter are prevalent today. Their advantage is that they have the possibility of hot sterilization. Fans circulating warm air can provide a uniform temperature distribution in the jacket and prevent the appearance of differently warm spots where moisture condensation may occur. In benchtop incubators, the chambers are heated by the heated floor and lid or through all six surfaces of the chamber. In this case, it is direct convection of heat from the heated metal plate to the petri dish.

After setting the temperature value in the incubator's menu, it is important to validate the actual temperature in the chamber by performing a set of temperature measurements with an independent calibrated thermometer. This can be done by placing sensitive thermologgers in different places within the chamber and by reading the results after a specific period of time. Temperature differences can exist between various locations inside the incubator, particularly in large-box incubators.[24] The validation report has to be prepared and kept with the incubator's documentation (Figure 2.3). The temperature recovery rates, described in the incubator's technical characteristics, should be validated too. Since there can be a considerable discrepancy between the recovery of temperature in the incubator's chamber and the incubated culture medium, particularly in classic large volume incubators,[5] it is recommended to measure the dynamics of temperature in both the atmosphere and culture medium after opening the incubator's door (see 2.6 Monitoring and Quality Control). Different laboratories use different culture dishes and volumes of culture media. For this reason, it is recommended that each laboratory makes its own set of temperature measurements to establish the actual temperature recovery rate in the dish.

2.5.2.4 Humidity

Most large incubators have some kind of humidification system to avoid the evaporation of culture media and, consequently, the increase of media osmolality. This can be a simple water reservoir positioned in the incubator from which the water slowly evaporates. Some large incubators have integrated pumps, which pass the water over a heater. After opening and closing the incubator door the water vapor quickly restores the relative humidity, particularly if the air is circulated by an integrated fan. Some benchtop and time lapse incubators achieve humidification by passing the gas through a water reservoir.

Constant humidity is needed in incubators for pre-incubation of culture media not overlaid with oil. However, even with oil overlay, if the petri dish with the same single-step medium is used for 5–6 days, its osmolality will increase and could negatively influence embryo development.[25] A humidified atmosphere may however increase the risk of contamination. The places where mold can occur are the water tank, rubber door seals, slots, and other hard-to-reach areas in the incubator, condensed moisture on the cooled walls, tubing system, fan, and perforated part of the gas sensors. The simpler the incubation chamber, the less likely is the occurrence of contamination. A humidified interior requires more frequent cleaning, disinfection, decontamination, or sterilization.

2.5.2.5 Air

The ambient air always enters the incubator's interior, no matter what gases are connected. In CO_2 incubators, the gas mixer uses as much as 95% of the ambient air and injects 5% of the CO_2 from the bottle. In O_2 incubators, the proportion of ambient air is lower, since the gas mixer uses most of the bottled gases (5% CO_2 and sufficient N_2 that only 5% O_2 is derived from ambient air). When a gas mixture is connected to the incubator, its interior is filled with 100% of the bottled gas. However, every time the incubator is opened, ambient air enters. As stated in section 2.3 Installation, the purity of bottled gas should be as high as possible (medical grade), to avoid the presence of toxic residues, in particular VOC, that may compromise embryo development.[26] However, in order to achieve high gas quality, it is advisable to attach special filters to the gas supply: high efficiency particulate absorption (HEPA) filters to reduce particles and to reduce VOCs. Modern benchtop incubators enable chamber atmosphere recirculation and its continuous HEPA filtration.

2.6 Monitoring and Quality Control

Provision of stable physicochemical parameters inside the incubators is essential to maintain quality and a safe embryo culture system. Here, it is important to distinguish between validation of the incubator, continuous monitoring of the parameters displayed, and independent monitoring performed with properly calibrated measuring instruments (quality control).

Validation is always performed before using the appliance by setting the desired parameter values and by checking them with independent measuring instruments. Frequently, the values shown on the incubator display and those shown on the measuring instruments differ. In this case, the incubator must be calibrated. After the reset is completed, enough time must lapse for the values to stabilize before remeasurement. This work should be done by a certified serviceman. Validation should be performed at least once a year. An example of temperature validation is shown in Figure 2.3.

Modern incubators have their own displays or are connected to an external computer equipped with data-logging software. This enables the continuous monitoring of set parameters and/or checking their past activity (Figure 2.4). Graphical representation of the measurements should be checked daily. Such an integrated quality control system, if the incubator comprises it, is effective if it can activate the alarm when the values go outside the limits of tolerance. The alarm should reach the responsible person. This can be done with a sound or light signal at the hospital emergency department or by calling the responsible person's mobile phone.

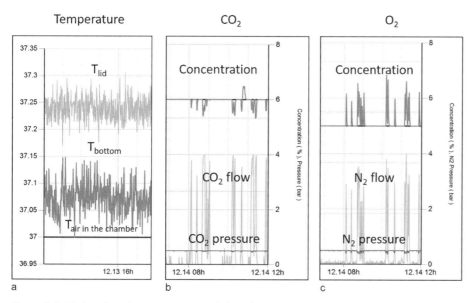

Figure 2.4 Display of continuous monitoring of physical parameters: **a.** temperature; **b.** CO_2, and **c.** O_2 concentrations. For color version of this figure. Please refer color plate section.

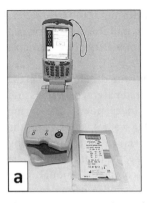
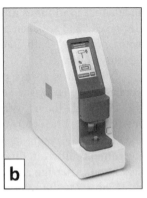

Figure 2.5 Measuring devices for measurement of: **a.** pH, and **b.** osmolality of incubated culture media. For color version of this figure. Please refer color plate section.

Despite integrated safety mechanisms to ensure constant conditions in the incubator, it is recommended to regularly perform independent measurements with calibrated measuring instruments, such as thermometers and gas concentration meters. In the author's laboratory, temperature, CO_2, and O_2 measurements are performed daily before the start of the clinical program, and the values are written on record forms.

In addition to a stable atmosphere within the incubator, it is important that the physicochemical parameters are stable in the embryo culture dishes. The measurement of temperature and gases in an incubator are simple compared to measurements in the culture medium itself. The values of physical parameters shown by the incubator display do not indicate that they have reached equilibrium in the culture medium. This effect is always delayed. Gases require some time to disperse into the medium and achieve the desired effect on its pH. Longer (5–6 days) incubation of culture media in a dry incubator can result in increased media osmolality. The pH and osmolality can be measured with specific measuring devices (Figure 2.5). Instruments for the measurement of temperature in the culture droplets must be adjusted with specific fine probes (Figure 2.6a). Modern incubators also have an integrated pH meter that continuously measures the pH of the media (Figure 2.6b). This technology uses an optical fluorescent measurement in combination with disposable sensors to monitor the pH of small volumes of culture medium. A very similar system (Hand O_2, Echo, Slovenia) has also been developed for continuous measurement of dissolved O_2 in the culture medium (Figure 2.6c,d), which is very important when ultra-low concentrations of O_2 are used for the embryo culture.

These instruments make it possible to monitor the dynamics of temperature, pH, and gases in the medium after the petri dish has been outside the incubator. Figure 2.7 shows the dynamics of the temperature during the conventional embryo assessment procedure when the petri dish is removed from the incubator, embryos moved to fresh medium and then evaluated under a microscope. A petri dish with culture medium was placed in a laminar flow hood for 2 minutes (the lid was removed from the dish for 1 minute). Although the temperature of the heating plate in laminar airflow hood was set to 40°C, the temperature in the petri dish dropped to almost 35°C. The recovery time was then dependent on the type of petri dish and the type of incubator. A 4-well dish required a much longer time to recover the temperature of the culture medium than a 35-mm petri dish. Benchtop incubators containing metal plates for specific petri dishes enabled direct contact of the dish with the plate. This helped to decrease the temperature recovery time. Small petri dishes with direct contact of their bottoms with the heating plate in benchtop incubators showed a superior temperature recovery time. To prevent a drop of the temperature in the culture medium, some petri dishes are designed without a ring on the bottom and allow direct contact with heating plates. Another option for recovering the temperature in Petri dishes as quickly as possible is to use metal coins in the incubators. The coins retain heat while opening the incubator door. When the petri dish is returned to the incubator, it is placed on a metal coin. The diameter of the coin is slightly smaller than the diameter of the petri dish, so the bottom of the petri dish is in direct contact with the surface of the coin.

The physical and chemical parameters are not the only factors to be checked within incubators. Despite the fact that working with embryo culture does not require completely aseptic conditions, regular checking for possible contamination of the incubator is essential. Embryo culture media are mostly covered with paraffin oil, which protects embryos relatively well and, at the same time, prevents the transfer of contamination from biological material to the incubator. Male ejaculates are not sterile and, despite proper sperm preparation for IVF, microorganisms can

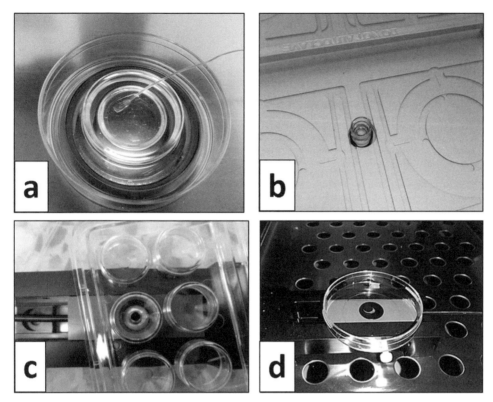

Figure 2.6 Continuous monitoring of physicochemical parameters in incubated culture media: **a.** fine temperature probe; **b.** integrated pH meter; **c.** and **d.** optical fluorescent measurement of dissolved O_2 in culture media. For color version of this figure. Please refer color plate section.

remain in the sample. Even though antibiotics are often added to the culture media, microorganisms can proliferate. Periodic swabs of the interior surfaces of incubators and classical testing for the growth of saprophytic bacterial and mold are routine inspections.

It is also recommended to include in the quality control system a follow up on success rates (fertilization, embryo development, implantation rates, live births rates) from each separate incubator.

2.7 Summary

Since embryos are cultured in incubators for several days, these devices represent the most important piece of equipment in any ART laboratory. Incubators have been technologically advanced since the beginning of ART. Numerous studies on the physiological requirements of embryos have shown that the constant temperature, osmolality, and pH of the media and the reduced O_2 concentration in the incubator atmosphere are crucial for normal embryo development. Although it is difficult to argue that more modern models of incubators could produce better clinical results, they nevertheless provide more stable physicochemical parameters during cultivation, thus avoiding additional stress for cells and embryos in vitro. Regardless of the type of incubator, all of them must be subject to the same standards of maintaining cleanliness, trouble-free operation, and constant control over their operation. Proper quality control of incubators requires some additional, regularly calibrated measuring instruments. It is recommended to measure physicochemical parameters not only inside the incubator, but especially in petri dishes with culture media. The stability of the measured values of these parameters, their recovery rate after incubator opening, and finally embryo quality and clinical outcomes are the main indicators of the quality of incubator performance and should be monitored for each individual incubator separately.

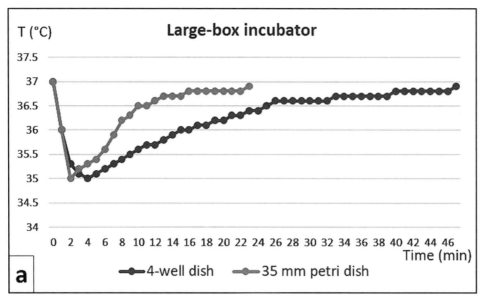

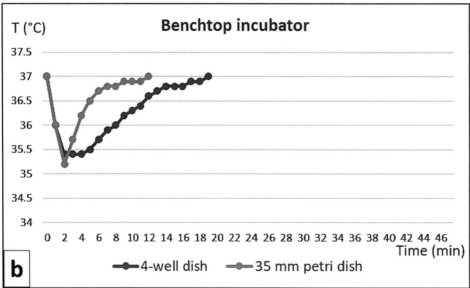

Figure 2.7 Recovery rate of the temperature of culture media after opening and closing of: **a.** large-box and **b.** benchtop incubators. For color version of this figure. Please refer color plate section.

References

1. Edwards RG. Test-tube babies, 1981. *Nature.* 1981;293:253–256.

2. Working group of ESHRE. Recommendations for good practice for the use of time-lapse technology. *Human Reprod Open.* 2020;(2)hoaa008.

3. Cohen J, Cairo 2018 Consensus Group. 'There is only one thing that is truly important in an IVF laboratory: everything' Cairo Consensus Guidelines on IVF Culture Conditions. *Reprod Biomed Online.* 2020;40:33–60.

4. Swain JE. Decisions for the IVF laboratory: comparative analysis of embryo culture incubators. *Reprod Biomed Online.* 2014;28:535–547.

5. Fujiwara M, Takahashi K, Izuno M, et al. Effect of micro-environment maintenance on embryo culture after in-vitro fertilization: comparison of top-load mini incubator and

conventional front-load incubator. *J Assist Reprod Genet.* 2007;24:5–9.

6. Gelo N, Kirinec G, Baldani DP, et al. Influence of human embryo cultivation in a classic CO$_2$ incubator with 20% oxygen versus benchtop incubator with 5% oxygen on live births: the randomized prospective trial. *Zygote.* 2019;27:131–136.

7. Lee M, Grazi R, Seifer D. Incorporation of the Cook K-Minc incubator and media system into the IVF lab: the future of IVF. *J Clin Embryol.* 2010;13:21–32.

8. Cruz M, Gadea B, Garrido N, et al. Embryo quality, blastocyst and ongoing pregnancy rates in oocyte donation patients whose embryos were monitored by time-lapse imaging. *J Assist Reprod Genet.* 2011;28:569–573.

9. Kirkegaard K, Hindkjaer JJ, Grondahl ML, Kesmodel US, Ingerslev HJ. A randomized clinical trial comparing embryo culture in a conventional incubator with a time-lapse incubator. *J Assist Reprod Genet.* 2012;29:565–572.

10. Hyslop L, Prathalingam N, Nowak L, et al. A novel isolator-based system promotes viability of human embryos during laboratory processing. *PLoS One* 2012; 7:e31010.

11. Mortimer D, Cohen J, Mortimer ST, et al. Cairo consensus on the IVF laboratory environment and air quality: report of an expert meeting. *Reprod Biomed Online.* 2018;36:658–674.

12. Chou J. Electrochemical sensors. In: *Hazardous Gas Monitors: A Practical Guide to Selection, Operation and Applications.* New York: McGraw Hill; 1999;27–35.

13. Swain JE. Media composition: pH and buffers. *Methods Mol Biol.* 2012;912:161–175.

14. Fischer B, Bavister BD. Oxygen tension in the oviduct and uterus of rhesus monkeys, hamsters and rabbits. *J Reprod Fertil.* 1993;99:673–679.

15. Ottosen LD, Hindkaer J, Husth M, Petersen DE, Kirk J, Ingerslev HJ. Observations on intrauterine oxygen tension measured by fibre-optic microsensors. *Reprod Biomed Online.* 2006;13:380–385.

16. Edwards RG, Steptoe PC, Purdy JM. Establishing full-term human pregnancies using cleaving embryos grown in vitro. *Br J Obstet Gynaecol.* 1980;87:737–756.

17. Lopata A, Johnston IWH, Hoult IJ, Speirs AL. Pregnancy following in-trauterine implantation of an embryo obtained by in vitro fertilization ofa preovulatory egg. *Fertil Steril.* 1980;33:117–120.

18. Testart J, Lassalle B, Frydman R. Apparatus for the in vitro fertilization and culture of human oocytes. *Fertil Steril.* 1982;38:372–375.

19. Kovačič B. Culture systems: low-oxygen culture. *Methods Mol Biol.* 2012;912:249–272.

20. Bontekoe S, Mantikou E, van Wely M, Seshadri S, Repping S, Mastenbroek S. Low oxygen concentrations for embryo culture in assisted reproductive technologies. *Cochrane Database Syst Rev.* 2012;11:CD008950.

21. ESHRE Guideline Group on Good Practice in IVF Labs, De los Santos MJ, Apter S, et al. Revised guidelines for good practice in IVF laboratories (2015). *Hum Reprod.* 2016;31:685–686.

22. Brinster RL. In vitro cultivation of mammalian ova. *Adv Biosci.* 1969;4:199–233.

23. Yedwab GA, Paz G, Homonnai TZ, David MP, Kraicer PF. The temperature, pH and partial pressure of oxygen in the cervix and uterus of women and uterus of rats during the cycle. *Fertil Steril.* 1976;27:304–309.

24. Walker MW, Butler JM, Higdon HL, Boone WR. Temperature variations within and between incubators – a prospective, observational study. *J Assist Reprod Genet.* 2013;30:1583–1585.

25. Swain JE. Controversies in ART: considerations and risks for uninterrupted embryo culture. *Reprod Biomed Online.* 2019;39:19–26.

26. Khoudja, RY, Xu Y, Li T, Zhou C. Better IVF outcomes following improvements in laboratory air quality. *J Assist Reprod Genet.* 2013; 30:69–76.

Consumables for the IVF Laboratory
Production and Validation, Quality Control, and Bioassays

Hubert Joris

3.1 Introduction

Since the birth of Louise Brown in 1978, IVF has evolved from a research-based environment to an established and regulated clinical treatment with around 2 million treatment cycles performed annually worldwide.

In the early days of IVF, success rates were relatively limited. Culture media and materials used within IVF clinics were homemade or developed for other purposes. While research on media for embryo culture increased from the 1950s, it is clear that media used in the infancy of IVF did not fully meet the needs of embryos to develop in vitro.[1] Before the implementation of disposable devices, sterilized glassware was used. For handling of oocytes or embryos as well as any micromanipulation technique applied, homemade pipettes were used. No information on endotoxin levels or other possible toxins present in these sterilized and homemade tools was available. Institutes with animal facilities were able to run a Mouse Embryo Assay on products while some others were using the Human Sperm Survival Assay as quality control. Many clinics, however, did not have the possibility to properly quality control the products used. There is evidence of effects on development from that period.[2,3]

While the role of a clinical IVF lab is to maintain viability of human gametes and embryos, it soon became evident that gametes and embryos have specific needs or sensitivities and that the products used did not always support requirements.

Development and commercialization of material and products for clinical ART started in the 1980s. At that time, regulation of ART was limited and classification of materials and products lacking.

While standard IVF is a relatively simple procedure, initially performed in a natural cycle, many new techniques have been implemented during the past four decades, adding increasing complexity to the laboratory and increasing the need for specific equipment and tools. Today, IVF labs are usually cleanroom-like environments where equipment and consumables, such as all types of media products, labware, or other single use devices, are fit for purpose, supporting success rates. Consumables used in the IVF laboratory are classified and approved by competent authorities before clinical use. This evolution has certainly contributed to today's success rates. The aim of this chapter is to describe specific aspects related to development and quality control of products used in clinical IVF on a daily basis, providing information to users to more critically assess product information provided by suppliers but also to challenge suppliers to provide more details on their efforts to provide products with maximum performance and safety.

3.2 Product Development for ART

Products used for treatment of patients are classified as medicinal products or medical devices. For many years it was unclear how products used in the human ART laboratory should be classified. Today, products used when handling human gametes and embryos are in many countries classified as medical device For the user, this means they should look for and use devices with the appropriate medical device approval. For the industry supplying products for IVF it means products must be developed, produced, and approved according to relevant market region regulations before they can be released on that specific market.

In Europe, medical device regulation has been harmonized since the early 1990s in the Medical Device Directive (MDD; Council Directive 93/42/EEC). The uncertainty regarding classification of products used in clinical ART resulted in use of products approved as in vitro diagnostic devices or without approval. To reduce confusion or misunderstanding regarding classification of products used in clinical ART, an EU guidance document (MEDDEV 2.2/4) was developed. Practically it means that products used when handling gametes or embryos are classified as medical devices.

To align with the developments in the medical field, the EU has recently updated the regulation for medical devices. This new Medical Device Regulation (MDR; Regulation (EU) 2017/745) will be enforced as of May 2020 and will replace the MDD and related guidance documents. For products currently approved under the MDD, manufacturers will have to comply with the MDR when the currently valid product CE certificate expires. (CE or Conformité Européenne means the product conforms to European legislation.) For their products to be CE approved, manufacturers of medical devices should also be ISO 13485 certified. This standard describes the quality system requirements for compliance of medical devices for regulatory approval. This means that manufacturers are audited for compliance with the ISO standard as well as for compliance of products with the general safety and performance requirements stipulated in the MDR.

Regulations on medical devices aim to guarantee safety and performance of products used. Authorities approve the products in the higher risk classes before they can be placed on the market and manufacturers are obliged to show that every batch of products released fulfils specifications. This is important for users as they rely on the suppliers of their products.

Development of medical devices is strictly regulated and MDR will further increase requirements and control from authorities on safety and performance of devices. Requirements for approval depend on the classification of the device. In the clinical IVF lab all classes of devices may be used (MDR Chapter V: Classification and Conformity Assessment). Even more than under MDD, post market surveillance will be important. Follow-up of products will be an important requirement and approvals will not be prolonged when evidence on safety and performance of products is not available.

Professionals from the field have suggested a path for development of products and implementation of new technologies.[4] The suggested path involves different phases starting with testing on animals followed by preclinical and clinical testing. Interestingly, when looking at the process for development of medical devices, the suggested path is in line with the development path for medical devices

described in the relevant ISO standards and regulatory documents.

Development of a new product includes different phases. Once research has provided enough information supporting development of a new product, the design control phase can be initiated. It is this phase that is scrutinized by relevant authorities when a manufacturer applies for regulatory approval. The design control phase includes different steps eventually leading to a final product (Figure 3.1) that can be transferred to the organization for production, testing, release, and distribution. All actions taken to go through this process are documented. Support from users can be required at different stages in this process and clinical investigations for development of new products usually take place during the design validation, which is among the final stages in the product development process (Figure 3.1). When all steps in the development process have been finalized and the documentation work for a product is completed, the approval process starts. Only when a product is approved by the competent authority can a new device become commercially available.

Twenty years ago, product development and product evaluation were very different. Safety and performance are now crucial criteria where evidence is required before a new product can be approved. This is for the benefit of the patient and gamete or embryo exposed to the devices. In practice, however, it also means that it will take several years before an idea can become an approved commercial product. When this path has been followed and a product becomes available, it is then up to the clinic to validate if the device meets clinic requirements or expectations for routine clinical use. When products are commercially available, local validation at the IVF clinic is performed according to the instructions for use. IVF clinics have their own procedures that may deviate from the manufacturer's instructions for use. Hence, validation by the clinic to collect evidence on the performance of a device is required before clinical implementation. The

3.3 Product Validation in the ART Laboratory

As mentioned, the approach during the late 1990s was that new products could be introduced easily. This was also a period where substantial progress in laboratory performance was made and people were quite open to implementing new products. The

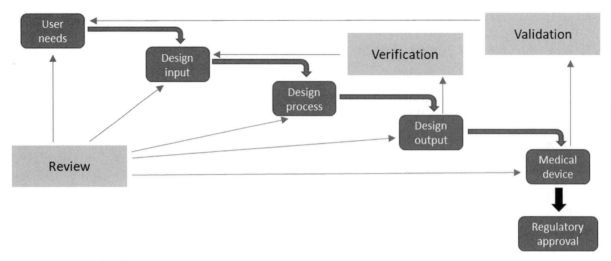

Figure 3.1 Process flow for medical device development. For color version of this figure. Please refer color plate section.

implementation of regulations, such as the directive on tissues and cells (2004/23/EC), and the increasing introduction of quality management systems mean that laboratories are now more prudent in the introduction of new devices or methods. Today, implementation of new devices involves validation to confirm the performance of the device in the IVF process of the clinic. In practice, this means that the introduction of a new device in clinical routine involves two independent validations, that is during the product development process by the manufacturer and the validation by the user in their own setting.

A clinic's quality management system normally describes how validation of a new device in clinical routine should be performed. Validation of a new device or method is not the same as a clinical investigation. While a clinical investigation aims to answer a scientific question, a validation aims to examine if performance of a device is according to expectations or requirements. Unlike a scientific study that may investigate a device as part of its development process, a validation aims to implement a product with adequate regulatory approval and therefore has different requirements regarding ethical approval and patient consent.

How to run a validation for implementation of a new device is a frequently asked question. Different aspects need to be considered.[5] The type of device affects how a validation can be performed. Validation of a time-lapse system is very different from introduction of a new medium for embryo transfer, a new denudation pipette or another method for oocyte vitrification. Each of them has specific aspects that must be taken into account. Another important criterion is how to run a comparison before introduction of a new product or method. If a device can be tested preclinically first, this should be the preferred track. This may, however, not always be possible. A comparison in the clinic can be made on sibling oocytes, or one can compare between patients. The differences between the two methods are listed in Table 3.1.

Besides the choice on how to set up a validation, the sample size is another aspect to consider. Ideally, a power calculation should be performed to determine the required number of cases but for validations this is usually not realistic. The possibility to run validations is largely affected by the size of the clinic. In any case, the sample size of a comparison should be large enough to give at least a good indication about the performance of a device. For example, sibling comparisons with fewer than six oocytes or zygotes per patient are difficult to compare. While it is always interesting to perform a statistical evaluation on the findings of a validation, interpretation should always be made with caution when limited sample sizes are involved. Significant differences from underpowered numbers can always be a chance finding. A comparison using a sibling design[6] and a patient comparison[7] are examples of sufficiently powered scientific studies comparing two products. For a validation, inclusion of at least 50 patients in a sibling design and 80–100 in a patient comparison can provide useful information on performance of a device.

Table 3.1 Aspects to consider in validation of new products or methods in the IVF laboratory

Sibling design	Patient comparison
■ Comparison on the same cohort	■ Comparison on different cohorts
■ Only patients with sufficient numbers of oocytes/zygotes can be included	■ All patients can be included
■ Avoids effect of patient factors	■ Patient factors can have important impact
■ Not possible to compare outcome except for single embryo transfer cases	■ Comparison of outcome possible but effect of sample size important
■ Affects workload due to duplication of treatment aspects	■ More demands on randomization to minimize possible patient effects
■ Very valuable for assessment of laboratory performance	■ Preferred when outcome data are important

Today, implementing a new medical device means a substantial amount of work to prove the performance and safety of a device. First there is the work done by the manufacturer before a product is approved. Proper validation at the clinic before general use adds to the information on performance of the device and will allow general use with limited risks of failure.

3.4 Quality Control on Medical Devices for ART

For the laboratory, an IVF procedure starts with collection of gametes and ends with the transfer of embryos, either fresh or after cryopreservation. Between the start and the end of a treatment, >100 devices may be used. While exposure to some devices may be only a few seconds, exposure to other devices can last several days. Nevertheless, the quality of each device contributes to the success of a treatment. Hence, the strength of a culture system is no stronger than the weakest link in the chain.

An IVF treatment involves a multidisciplinary approach where collaboration between the clinic and laboratory is required. The laboratory aims to create an environment where fertilization can take place and embryos develop in the best possible conditions. Physical and chemical conditions are important aspects in providing an optimal environment.[8] Optimization of temperature and the gas phase contributes substantially. Other aspects are the consumables that gametes and embryos are in contact with. Gametes and embryos are in direct contact with media and culture dishes and have the longest contact time with these products. This can partly explain why these products are often suspected first in case of changes in results. Although gametes and embryos are not in direct contact with it, oil can also be harmful and affect results.[9] Besides, any device used can potentially exert a negative effect, independent from its exposure time or whether there is direct or indirect contact. Therefore, quality control (QC) should be equally strict for any device used.

Results of IVF have improved continuously over the years. Part of this can certainly be attributed to increased quality of devices used. As mentioned in 3.1 Introduction, in the early days of IVF no products fitting the exact purpose existed and no adequate QC was performed before using devices clinically. Evidence on suboptimal quality of products used in the IVF lab has been published.[10,11]

While gametes and embryos have specific needs, they also have specific sensitivities, imposing specific requirements on products designed and produced for use in clinical ART. It is essential that QC tests identify products of suboptimal quality. Depending on the type of product, different QC tests are used. Common tests for most devices are for sterility and endotoxin, as well as bioassays.

Exposure of medical devices to gametes or embryos as part of a QC program is a logical approach for these types of devices, and so the use of bioassays for human ART was suggested in the early days of IVF.[12] Sperm cells of different species have been used in bioassays.[13] Today, a Human Sperm Survival Assay (HSSA) is most common.[10] For tests including embryos, the Mouse Embryo Assay (MEA) is used.[11,14] Other types of cell lines have been suggested in the past but have not proven to be equally effective as MEA.

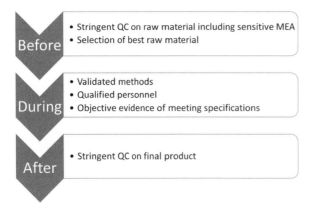

Before
- Stringent QC on raw material including sensitive MEA
- Selection of best raw material

During
- Validated methods
- Qualified personnel
- Objective evidence of meeting specifications

After
- Stringent QC on final product

Figure 3.2 Proposed flow for production of medical devices for ART, including raw material selection. For color version of this figure. Please refer color plate section.

Users receive a Certificate of Analysis (COA) listing important specifications of the product and the results of QC testing on the final product. The COA lists specifications considered important for the device and results from the QC testing must be within the predefined specifications. These specifications can be dimensions or other features that are relevant for the product. For media products, pH and osmolality is often included. Furthermore, results on sterility, endotoxins, and bioassays are listed whenever applicable.

For most products, the bioassay of choice is an MEA but for products exposed to sperm cells only, it can be an HSSA. The QC tests listed on the COA have been specified during the development process and are thus part of the suppliers' quality management system. This testing is performed on the final product. A failure in final product testing, that is when any of the parameters listed on the COA is out of specification, does not allow release of the product which, in a worst-case scenario, can have an impact on treatment of patients. In the late 1980s and early 1990s when commercialization of products for IVF started, sometimes a company could not provide product due to failing QC. This can be overcome by making appropriate QC testing measures during the production process, including for incoming raw materials.

This testing on raw materials can also include MEAs.[14] A recent inquiry on manufacturer practices for QC testing showed that only a limited number of manufacturers perform MEAs on incoming material.[15] Such testing has, however, important benefits. When testing raw materials before release to the production process, raw materials meeting requirements

can be selected. Such a selection process, together with a controlled production process and final product testing supports performance and safety of devices (Figure 3.2). Raw materials can be, e.g., metal for production of aspiration needles, glass for production of micromanipulation or denudation pipettes, pellets of plastic raw material used for production of labware, oil, chemicals used for production of media as well as any product in contact with the raw materials during production processes. Including such raw material testing and selection requires extensive effort but is also efficient as it will exclude inferior raw materials, some already being critical for success in IVF, at an early time point, thereby minimizing risks in quality issues.

One such example is oil used for overlay. Oil is continuously used in human IVF and has important advantages. Oil should be considered a critical product taking into account the evidence on its effects on embryo development. The aforementioned testing of raw material can play an important role in finding product of sufficient quality. Otsuki et al showed that different oils released for use in clinical ART had different levels of peroxidation that, depending on storage conditions, increased over time in a number of products.[16] Based on the findings, some of these oils would result in a toxic product during storage. Except for a selection in the type of oil used, it has been documented that modifications in culture protocols, including 1-cell MEA,[17] using different strain of mice[18] and adding cell counts as endpoint of an MEA,[14,19] adds to the identification of good quality oil. Performing such testing on raw material increases the likelihood to produce high-quality products but also minimizes batch-to-batch variation.

Another critical component that is used in media products is albumin. While albumin solutions are normally registered as medicinal products and can be applied safely in patients, not all albumin is safe for use in human IVF.[20] Albumin is produced from pooled blood provided by donors. Purity of albumin solutions is around 98 % and contains a number of other components[21] that may have a positive or a negative effect. Albumin solutions also contain stabilizers that have a concentration dependent effect.[22] Taken this information together, it seems obvious that preselection of albumin raw material is an important contributor to final product quality.

Also the raw material used to produce plastic labware is very important. Different types of plastics are used and different quality levels of the raw materials exist. Again, testing and selection of raw materials meeting requirements supports production of a high-quality product.

Production processes involve all types of materials that come in contact with the product being made. This may also be a potential cause of contamination or toxicity. Hence, full control of production processes benefits from assessment of the quality and safety of the materials used. Specifically for labware, this is important as different chemicals may be used to optimize production but those components are not necessarily embryo-friendly. This is another example where thorough control supports product quality.

Disposables used in clinical ART are sterile. Assessment of sterility is one of the tests performed on the final product. Different procedures for sterilization resulting in different levels of sterility are used. The choice of sterilization method largely depends on the type of product. Among others, sterilization can be done using heat, radiation, gas or filtration. Sterilization of devices is performed according to the relevant applicable ISO standards. Devices made of metal, plastic or glass can usually be sterilized using techniques providing a Sterility Assurance Level (SAL) of SAL 10^{-6}. For media products used in ART this is not possible. Media products are filtered aseptically. This process can provide a sterility level that is SAL 10^{-3}. Sterility tests are part of final product testing and typically take 2 weeks to obtain results.

Any device can therefore not be released during the first weeks following production.

Concerns have been raised regarding possible effects of sterilization processes on quality of the sterilized devices, possibly resulting in changes of features or characteristics of the device or toxicities for gametes or embryos.[23,24] The sterilization method is chosen to avoid possible effects on features or characteristics of the device. Sterilization processes are standardized and compliance with these standards is documented and reviewed by competent authorities. However, variation in doses applied for sterilization is possible and must be considered to minimize possible effects of the sterilization process while still obtaining sterile product. For filtration methods, sufficient rinsing of filters before starting the filtration process and aliquot into vials or bottles helps in minimizing possible negative effects of the filters.[24]

Depending on the method of sterilization, a consequence of the sterilization process can be release of VOCs. Since the product is packed before sterilization, VOCs derived from the sterilization process remain inside the package. When opening a package with sterilized product, it may smell. Historical practice has been to off-gas materials after opening the package and for some time before use.

Performing MEAs on the final product should also mean it is done after sterilization. In that case, it will also control for possible effects of the sterilization process. Figure 3.3 shows the results of an MEA

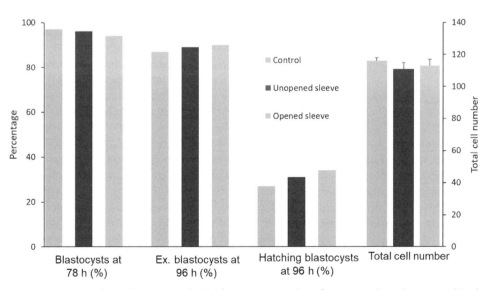

Figure 3.3 MEA results on labware immediately after opening or 7 days after opening. For color version of this figure. Please refer color plate section.

Figure 3.4 ISO symbol for single use. For color version of this figure. Please refer color plate section.

on a sterilized product immediately after opening of package and after off-gassing for 7 days. Embryo development and cell number is similar between control and sterilized dishes with or without off-gassing, showing that proper control of sterilization processes, even if labware packages may smell upon opening, does not result in toxic effects.

All sterile devices have an expiry date. For products such as needles, pipettes or labware this is typically 3 years from production. For media or oil this is usually much shorter, around 6–8 weeks. Shelf life is also controlled by competent authorities and a manufacturer has to show objective evidence to allow for the proposed shelf lives. This evidence is provided by stability studies where relevant tests are performed at predefined frequencies and have to show results within specification for each product. Similar evidence is required in cases when multiple use may be possible. This may be the case for media products. Presence of the appropriate ISO symbol regarding single use (Figure 3.4) on the label of a device is mandatory and informs the user if a bottle containing medium may be used over several days or not. The instructions will then state how long a bottle can be used following opening.

While devices may be sterile, this does not necessarily mean they are endotoxin-free. Endotoxins are membrane fragments from gram-negative bacteria. Sterilization may thus result in generation of endotoxins. Presence of endotoxins can affect results of ART in humans[25] and in animal species.[26] Therefore, testing for endotoxins is important and today this is done using the Limulus Amoebocyte Lysate assay (LAL-test). Besides testing on a final product, testing of raw materials is supportive in selecting such materials free from microbiological contamination. Bioburden testing on provides information about such contamination. Avoiding contaminated raw material decreases risks for contamination during the production process.

Manufacturers have control over the product until it is shipped to customers. Wherever necessary, conditions of shipment are also validated to guarantee

appropriate conditions during transport. This is done according to applicable ISO standards. Manufacturers have, however, no control over a product once it arrives at the end users. While the manufacturer provides information about storage and use of devices, meeting these requirements is the responsibility of the user. To minimize temperature variation and allow proper control, use of medical grade refrigerators is highly recommended for all products requiring cold storage.

Bioassays are an important part of QC testing for devices used in ART. The HSSA and MEA are both commonly used but the value of these tests has been questioned. Testing of medical devices for biological safety involves several types of bioassays. The relevant ISO standard describes the tests that have to be performed during product development as part of the evidence for biological safety of a product. Whenever applicable, MEA and HSSA are performed routinely for each batch of final product. However, although they are important QC tests for medical devices in human ART, MEA, and HSSA are not yet standardized. Recently, efforts to improve this have been proposed (https://www.fda.gov/regulatory-information/search-fda-guidance-documents/mouse-embryo-assay-assisted-reproduction-technology-devices).

3.5 Mouse Embryo Assay

It is obvious from the information above that the MEA can be a crucial test in providing quality products. It is generally accepted in the field that medical devices used in human ART undergo MEA testing. Communications with embryologists, however, also shows that knowledge about the MEA is limited. Similar to a clinical lab, also an MEA involves numerous variables that may have an effect on the result of the bioassay. These variables include embryo density (number of embryos per volume of medium), protein supplementation, and gas phase. Additionally, the strain of mice and the developmental stage at the start of the assay have an effect. As well as the conditions mentioned, the endpoint of a MEA can differ. Blastocyst formation is the most common end point. However, there is evidence that this may not be the best endpoint to identify embryo viability.[27] Since cell counts are a better indication of embryo viability, this is a more informative endpoint of an MEA.

Table 3.2 Possible questions to consider to learn more about MEA

Which bioassay is relevant for the product?
How is the test product exposed to the sperm cells or mouse embryos? • For how long? • Is there any treatment of or addition to the media exposed to the test item? • Are all parts of a device included in the test?
How many embryos are used for one MEA?
Is culture individual or in group? In case of group culture, what is the embryo density (embryo per medium volume)? For single culture, what is the medium volume?
Is there a control group in each test?
What is the developmental stage at the start of the MEA?
Except when testing specific culture media, which test medium is used to grow the embryos? Does the test medium contain albumin?
What is the culture environment (gas phase) to culture the embryos?
What is the endpoint of the MEA?
In case of blastocyst formation, after how many hours is the final assessment of development?

Last but not least is also the exposure of the test device to the mouse embryos. It sounds logical that exposure time to the test item is in line with its use. For devices other than media, the device should be exposed to media in which embryos are then cultured without any additional dilution or supplementation of the medium after the exposure. Lack of standardization, however, means that today there is no control over the way products are exposed or culture is performed.

Considering all the information available pointing to improved sensitivity of the MEA with optimized test conditions and cell counts as the endpoint increased attention from users is warranted to challenge suppliers to provide detailed information about test conditions. Evidence for differences in test conditions between suppliers of medical devices used in human ART is available.[15, 28] Table 3.2 shows a list of questions one may consider when aiming to understand more about MEA or HSSA tests performed on devices used in ART. The recent FDA document with guidelines on how to perform MEA is a step forward but the current proposed methodology does not include aspects where others showed a beneficial effect on detecting toxicity for mouse embryos.[17, 18, 19]

3.6 Summary

Today, an IVF treatment cycle involves numerous products that are classified as medical devices in most countries. Development and production of medical devices is strictly regulated and updated regulations will further increase the requirements for manufacturers to provide evidence on performance and safety of their devices. Users of these devices have a responsibility to validate introduction of new devices and this can be done in different ways. Independent from the way a comparison is designed, sufficient sample size is important and interpretation of statistical findings should be made with caution in case of insufficient power.

Quality testing of devices is important. Taking into account the specific requirements gametes and embryos have, use of appropriately performed bioassays is important. So far, no standardization of bioassays specifically for IVF is in place and there are differences in the way MEA is performed. Considering details of the MEA helps in deciding on the products to use.

Over the years, the quality of devices used in ART has improved. Today, products are fit for purpose and clinics have tools to evaluate the choice of product to use for patient treatment. Further optimization of product quality together with efforts from the field to improve results will support further improvement of results. However, no matter what effort is made, a culture system is only as strong as the weakest link and, therefore, every little detail counts and is equally important.

References

1. Bolton VN, Hawes SM, Taylor CT, Parsons JH. Development of spare human preimplantation embryos in vitro: an analysis of the correlations among gross morphology, cleavage rates, and development to the blastocyst. *J In Vitro Fert Embryo Transf.* 1989;6:30–35.

2. Ray BD, McDermott A, Wardle PG, et al. In vitro fertilization: fertilization failure due to toxic catheters. *J In Vitro Fert Embryo Transf.* 1987;4:58–61.

3. Hinduja I, Peter J, Menezes J. Instrument failure in in vitro fertilization: a case report. *J In Vitro Fert Embryo Transf.* 1985;2:108–109.

4. Harper J, Magli MC, Lundin K, Barratt CL, Brison D. When and how should new technology be introduced into the IVF laboratory? *Hum Reprod.* 2012;27:303–313.

5. Provoost V, Tilleman K, D'Angelo A, et al. Beyond the dichotomy: a tool for distinguishing between experimental, innovative and established treatment. *Hum Reprod.* 2014;29:413–417.

6. Hardarson T, Bungum M, Conaghan J, et al. Noninferiority, randomized, controlled trial comparing embryo development using media developed for sequential or undisturbed culture in a time–lapse setup. *Fertil Steril.* 2015;104:1452–1459.e1–4.

7. Kleijkers SH, Mantikou E, Slappendel E, et al. Influence of embryo culture medium (G5 and HTF) on pregnancy and perinatal outcome after IVF: a multicenter RCT. *Hum Reprod.* 2016;31:2219–2230.

8. Wale PL, Gardner DK. The effects of chemical and physical factors on mammalian embryo culture and their importance for the practice of assisted human reproduction. *Hum Reprod Update.* 2016;22:2–22.

9. Otsuki J, Nagai Y, Chiba K. Peroxidation of mineral oil used in droplet culture is detrimental to fertilization and embryo development. *Fertil Steril.* 2007;88:741–743.

10. Nijs M, Franssen K, Cox A, Wissmann D, Ruis H, Ombelet W. Reprotoxicity of intrauterine insemination and in vitro fertilization–embryo transfer disposables and products: a 4–year survey. *Fertil Steril.* 2009;92:527–535.

11. Punt–van der Zalm JP, Hendriks JC, Westphal JR, Kremer JA, Teerenstra S, Wetzels AM. Toxicity testing of human assisted reproduction devices using the mouse embryo assay. *Reprod Biomed Online.* 2009;18:529–535.

12. Ackerman SB, Stokes GL, Swanson RJ, Taylor SP, Fenwick L. Toxicity testing for human in vitro fertilization programs. *J In Vitro Fert Embryo Transf.* 1985;2:132–137.

13. Bavister BD, Andrews JC. A rapid sperm motility bioassay procedure for quality–control testing of water and culture media. *J In Vitro Fert Embryo Transf.* 1988;5:67–75.

14. Gardner DK, Reed L, Linck D, Sheehan C, Lane M. Quality control in human in vitro fertilization. *Semin Reprod Med.* 2005;23:319–324.

15. Delaroche L, Oger P, Genauzeau E. Embryotoxicity testing of IVF disposables: how do manufacturers test? *Hum Reprod.* 2020;35:283–292.

16. Otsuki J, Nagai Y, Chiba K. Damage of embryo development caused by peroxidized mineral oil and its association with albumin in culture. *Fertil Steril.* 2009;91:1745–1749.

17. Hughes PM, Morbeck DE, Hudson SB, Fredrickson JR, Walker DL, Coddington CC. Peroxides in mineral oil used for in vitro fertilization: defining limits of standard quality control assays. *J Assist Reprod Genet.* 2010;27:87–92.

18. Khan Z, Wolff HS, Fredrickson JR, Walker DL, Daftary GS, Morbeck DE. Mouse strain and quality control testing: improved sensitivity of the mouse embryo assay with embryos from outbred mice. *Fertil Steril.* 2013;99:847–854.e2.

19. Ainsworth AJ, Fredrickson JR, Morbeck DE. Improved detection of mineral oil toxicity using an extended mouse embryo assay. *J Assist Reprod Genet.* 2017;34:391–397.

20. Morbeck DE, Paczkowski M, Fredrickson JR. Composition of protein supplements used for human embryo culture. *J Assist Reprod Genet.* 2014;31:1703–1711.

21. Dyrlund TF, Kirkegaard K, Poulsen ET. Unconditioned commercial embryo culture media contain a large variety of non–declared proteins: a comprehensive proteomics analysis. *Hum Reprod.* 2014;29:2421–2430.

22. Fredrickson J, Krisher R, Morbeck DE. The impact of the protein stabilizer octanoic acid on embryonic development and fetal growth in a murine model. *J Assist Reprod Genet.* 2015;32:1517–1524.

23. Schiewe MC, Schmidt PM, Bush M, Wildt DE. Toxicity potential of absorbed–retained ethylene oxide residues in culture dishes on embryo development in vitro. *J Anim Sci.* 1985;60:1610–1618.

24. Harrison KL, Sherrin DA, Hawthorne TA, Breen TM, West GA, Wilson LM. Embryotoxicity of micropore filters used in liquid sterilization. *J In Vitro Fert Embryo Transf.* 1990;7:347–350.

25. Nagata Y, Shirakawa K. Setting standards for the levels of endotoxin in the embryo

culture media of human in vitro fertilization and embryo transfer. *Fertil Steril*. 1996;65:614–619.

26. Dubin NH, Bornstein DR, Gong Y. Use of endotoxin as a positive (toxic) control in the mouse embryo assay. *J Assist Reprod Genet*. 1995;12:147–152.

27. Lane M, Gardner DK. Differential regulation of mouse embryo development and viability by amino acids. *J. Reprod. Fertil.* 1997; 109:153–164.

28. Janssens R, Verheyen G, Cortvrindt R. A review of commercial MEA testing and plea for informative MEA certificates of analysis. Abstracts of the 10th Biennial Conference of Alpha, Scientists in Reproductive Medicine, 9–11 May 2014, Antalya, Turkey. *Reprod Biomed Online*. 2014;28(suppl 1) S2.

Chapter 4

Embryo Metabolism and What Does the Embryo Need?

Paula Vergaro and Roger G. Sturmey

4.1 Embryo Metabolism: An Overview

The embryo is a dynamic structure that can be affected by the interaction with the surrounding environment. During its journey through the female reproductive tract from fertilization to implantation, the embryo undergoes numerous biochemical and physiological changes which are essential for a successful reproductive outcome. During successive cleavage rounds, the embryo increases in cell number, switches from maternal to embryonic genome control (embryonic genome activation; EGA) and forms cell–cell junctions. This coincides with the cells flattening and compacting at the morula stage (Coticchio et al., 2019). At the final stage of the preimplantation period, the blastomeres differentiate to form the trophectoderm and the inner cell mass cell lineages. The blastocyst undergoes remarkable events in preparation for implantation and establishment of pregnancy, including initiation of overall growth, significant rise in transcriptional activity, increased protein synthesis, and active Na$^+$/K$^+$ ATPase activity in the trophectoderm leading to the formation of the blastocoel cavity (reviewed by Smith & Sturmey, 2013). The blastocyst also improves homeostatic regulatory mechanisms, including defense against oxidative damage (Lane & Gardner, 2000). These changes are energy dependent, and therefore underpinned by specific metabolic pathways. Disruptions in energy production during the preimplantation period are related to embryonic developmental impairment and reduced fetal viability post-transfer (Gardner, 1998; Lane & Gardner, 2005b). For these reasons, metabolism is considered a key determinant of embryo competence and viability.

As in other cells, metabolism in the embryo aims to provide energy (mainly by producing ATP, NADH, and FADH$_2$) to maintain normal cellular function as well as to provide precursors for the macromolecule synthesis (Figure 4.1). Embryo energy metabolism follows a generally accepted pattern of progressing from being relatively quiescent during cleavage to an overall boost of oxygen and glucose consumption as well as lactate production at the blastocyst stage (Leese, 2012). The cleavage stage embryo uses pyruvate as a major source of energy, which is obtained from glycolysis or the external environment and consumed at all stages of preimplantation development (Lewis & Sturmey, 2015).

After compaction and blastocyst formation, glycolysis becomes prevalent, leading to rising glucose consumption rates (Leese, 2012).

Carbohydrates and energy metabolism have long been the focus of attention while studying embryo development, but there is now compelling evidence that other components, including amino acids and lipids, are crucial for correct development of the embryo during the preimplantation period.

Embryo metabolism is mostly quantified as the uptake and release of different compounds into the culture medium (Leese & Barton, 1984; Guerif et al., 2013). Despite the inherent variability in metabolism between embryos, viable embryos appear to share the feature of "lower" levels of metabolic activity compared to those that are nonviable. This was elegantly summarized by Leese in 2002 (Leese, 2002) which lead to the "Quiet Embryo Hypothesis." This was refined further to include molecular determinants leading to these distinct phenotypes (Baumann et al., 2007), the concept of a "quiet range" (Leese et al., 2007) and different categories of quietness (Leese et al., 2008a). The most recent update of the initial hypothesis includes the concept of a "Goldilocks zone" or "lagom," which refers to the "just-right" range within which those embryos with maximum developmental potential are located. This would imply a minimum threshold to maintain energy homeostasis and an upper limit to maximize cellular metabolism performance (Leese et al., 2016, Leese et al., 2019).

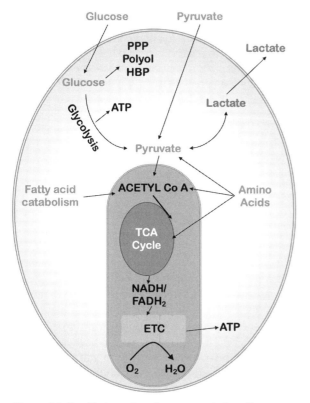

Figure 4.1 Simplified overview of energy metabolism. Glucose can enter the cell and take part in a variety of pathways; however, only glycolysis can generate ATP. The end product of glycolysis is pyruvate. This may be converted into lactate and excreted by the cell, or the pyruvate may be taken into the mitochondria and converted into acetyl Co A. Pyruvate itself may be taken up by the cell and used directly to make acetyl Co A. Acetyl Co A can also by synthesized by fatty acid catabolism or conversion of a number of amino acids. Acetyl Co A feeds into the TCA cycle which occurs in the mitochondrial matrix and produces the electronic carriers NADH and FADH2. These transport electrons to Complex 1 and Complex 2 respectively of the electron transport chain (ETC). The final reaction of the electron transport chain is the phosphorylation of ADP to make ATP and the reduction of molecular oxygen to water. This is the major cellular consumer of oxygen and is the reason that measurement of oxygen consumption is a good marker of mitochondrial activity. For color version of this figure. Please refer color plate section.

4.2 What Does an Embryo Need, and Why?

As previously described, the embryo changes dramatically from fertilization to implantation as it moves from the fallopian tube to the uterus. Those changes are critical for embryo development and are driven largely by the energy requirements at each stage, which mirror ATP demands. In order to satisfy these needs, the embryo adapts its energy metabolism and uses a variety of sources from those present in the

physiological environment to which it is sequentially exposed (Gardner et al., 1996). The mammalian oviduct and uterine fluids are composed of a myriad of factors secreted by epithelial cells or derived from blood plasma, including energy substrates traditionally added to culture media (i.e., glucose, lactate, and pyruvate) as well as albumin, glycoproteins, amino acids, growth factors, and electrolytes (e.g., potassium and bicarbonate) (Leese, 1988; Aguilar & Reyley, 2005; Leese et al., 2008b; Cheong et al., 2013; Kermack et al., 2015). In vitro culture must replicate those conditions as closely as possible in order to reduce the stress that the embryo suffers when taken from its physiological environment (Gardner & Leese, 1990).

4.2.1 Energy Substrates or Carbohydrates

Glucose, lactate, and pyruvate are major nutrients for ATP production and normal cellular development. Apart from energy sources, these molecules play a variety of important roles: glucose is involved in biosynthetic processes (e.g., nucleic acid and protein synthesis) and acts as a cell signaling factor. Glucose is also required for embryos to express specific nutrient transporters, whose activity, in turn, regulates intracellular pH and the reactive oxygen species-mediated stress response (Leese, 2012). It has been suggested that at time of implantation, lactate facilitates trophoblast invasion by lowering the pH and promoting uterine tissue degradation as well as by acting as a signaling factor to induce endometrial immune and vascular responses (Gardner, 2015). Pyruvate appears to be essential to overcome the so-called "2-cell block" in mice and must be present in a specific time frame, as shown by Nagaraj et al., (2017). They demonstrated that EGA occurs only when the enzyme pyruvate dehydrogenase locates to the nucleus at the 2-cell stage in mice or 4-cell stage in human, for which the presence of pyruvate is required (Nagaraj et al., 2017). When pyruvate is not present, the normal phenotype can be rescued by precursors of pyruvate, a-ketoglutarate, and arginine. This key observation expands on the traditional view of metabolism beyond the provision of energy and indicates molecular regulatory roles for metabolic processes.

4.2.2 Amino Acids

Protein synthesis is low during early stages of embryo development and increases at the blastocyst stage,

---

Box 4.1 Essential vs Nonessential amino

The 20 common protein-encoding amino acids are commonly placed into two convenient groups: *essential* or *nonessential*. This categorization is based on whether amino acids can be made by the body from other substrates (i.e., nonessential) or whether they must be provided from the diet, because they cannot be synthesized de novo in sufficient quantities to satisfy needs (i.e., essential). This is an unfortunate terminology since it implies that some amino acids are not essential; however, all of the 20 amino acids are components of protein.

Typically, eight amino acids are considered essential – leucine, isoleucine, valine, threonine, methionine, phenylalanine, tryptophan, and lysine. These distinctions are based on knowledge of whole body nutrition of adults.

To complicate matters further, a further seven amino acids – arginine, histidine, glycine, tyrosine, glutamine, cysteine, and proline – are essential for children, since de novo synthesis is insufficient to satisfy demand. These are often termed *conditionally essential*.

Thus, applying the concept of essential and non-essential amino acids to the embryo may not be truly representative of the needs of the developing embryo in vitro.

---

concomitant with embryo growth. However, exogenous amino acids supplied by culture media are incorporated into proteins during the early preimplantation stages, which justifies their wide presence in current culture media (Epstein & Smith, 1973; Summers & Biggers, 2003). Often, amino acids are classified into two groups – so called *essential* and *non-essential*. The origin of these terms come from whole body physiology, and relates to whether they can be synthesized de novo or whether they need to be taken up from dietary sources – see Box 4.1 for further explanation. The aspects of amino acid turnover in relation with embryo development and supplementation in culture media have been comprehensively reviewed by Sturmey et al. (2008). Apart from their classical function as building blocks for protein synthesis (Crosby et al., 1988), amino acids play a variety of key roles in the preimplantation embryo. They may act as chelators and antioxidants (Suzuki et al., 2007), regulate the intracellular pH (Edwards et al., 1998a), and serve as organic osmolytes (Dawson & Baltz, 1997). Amino acids also mediate important signaling processes for development and implantation (reviewed by Van Winkle et al., 2006); e.g. it has been suggested, that leucine and arginine regulate trophoblast motility at the time of implantation in mice (Gonzalez et al., 2012). Furthermore, amino acids provide precursors for nucleotide, GTP, and NAD+ synthesis (Leese et al., 1993) and can regulate carbohydrate metabolism (Lane & Gardner, 2005a; Mitchell et al., 2009).

Human embryos show stage-specific patterns of amino acid release and consumption (Houghton et al., 2002; Brison et al., 2004; Stokes et al., 2007) and display general patterns of glutamine, leucine, and arginine consumption as well as alanine release throughout the preimplantation period (Houghton et al., 2002; Brison et al., 2004; Stokes et al., 2007). Given the importance of amino acid functions in embryo development, many studies have researched the possibility of using them as predictors of IVF success. Viable embryos showed a different metabolic profile from that of nonviable embryos in different species, including humans (Houghton et al., 2002; Brison et al., 2004; Orsi & Leese, 2004a; Humpherson et al., 2005; Sturmey et al., 2009). Interestingly, the metabolic signature has also been related to embryo sex (Sturmey et al., 2010; Gardner et al., 2011) as well as to DNA integrity, genetic health and assembly of trophectoderm cell junctions (Eckert et al., 2007; Picton et al., 2010; Sturmey et al., 2010). The amino acid profile is therefore an indirect evidence of the roles mentioned above, giving a snapshot of the physiological status of the embryo.

4.2.3 Fatty Acids

In addition to exogenous nutrients, embryos also utilize some endogenous energy stores, such as fatty acids. Fatty acids are constituents of lipids and part of all cell membranes. In addition, fatty acids are stored in cells as cytoplasmic hydrophobic lipid droplets, essentially formed by a neutral core of triglyceride and cholesterol esters coated by a phospholipid monolayer and proteins (Walther & Farese, 2012). The amount and distribution of lipid droplets is species specific. Pig, cattle, and sheep oocytes and embryos show significant levels of fatty acids (Coull et al., 1998; Ferguson & Leese, 1999; McEvoy et al., 2000; Sturmey & Leese, 2003; Leroy et al., 2005; Sturmey et al., 2006; Sudano et al., 2011), which are responsible for their characteristic dark appearance compared to those of mice or human, which have low and moderate lipid content, respectively (Matorras et al., 1998; Haggarty et al., 2006; Bradley et al., 2016). Fatty acids are important sources of energy for preimplantation embryo development, and the importance of fatty acid for embryo development has been demonstrated in species with lower lipid content, such as mice and human. Using a forced selective autophagy of lipid droplets system, it has been demonstrated that mouse embryos require endogenous lipids to develop, showing decreased triglyceride levels and developmental impairment when the number of lipid droplets was reduced (Tatsumi et al., 2018).

4.3 How Does the Embryo Utilize Nutrients?

Energy metabolism is compartmentalized in the cytosol (glycolysis) or the mitochondria (TCA cycle, β-oxidation, and oxidative phosphorylation) of living cells (Figure 4.1). In the egg, pyruvate and lactate are produced from glucose by the cumulus cells (Leese & Barton, 1985; Gardner & Leese, 1990; Gardner et al., 1996). In the cleavage stage embryo, before compaction, the majority of ATP is produced through mitochondrial oxidation of pyruvate, as well as low levels of lactate (from the 2-cell stage) and certain amino acids. Around 85–90% of ATP in pre-compaction embryos is derived through oxidative phosphorylation (Thompson et al., 1996; Sturmey & Leese, 2003).

It is noteworthy that despite oxidative metabolism being the main source of ATP during the pre-compaction period, overall oxygen consumption rates remain low until the blastocyst stage, when energy demands increase (Houghton et al., 1996; Goto et al., 2018). Indeed, postimplantation oxygen consumption rates of human embryos are similar to those of pre-compaction stages, highlighting the high energy demands accompanying blastocyst formation and largely derived from the Na^+/K^+ ATPase activity (Houghton et al., 2003). Oxidation of pyruvate through the TCA cycle is the main source of energy production, but other substrates, such as amino acids, can be incorporated into this metabolic pathway. In

particular, glutamine appears important for embryo development in cattle, mice, pig, and human (Devreker et al., 1998; Steeves & Gardner, 1999; Houghton et al., 2002; Brison et al., 2004; Rezk et al., 2004; Chen et al., 2018).

Accompanying the rise in energy demands at the blastocyst stage is a fall in ATP levels as it is rapidly consumed, and a simultaneous increase in AMP levels. An important aspect of glucose metabolism in the blastocyst is that, in the presence of oxygen, they do not oxidize all the glucose but rather convert part of it to lactate. This phenomenon is known as aerobic glycolysis and mirrors the so-called Warburg effect, which appears to be a feature of rapidly dividing cells, such as cancer cells (Warburg, 1956; Redel et al., 2012). The parallels between the metabolism of embryos and cancer cells have been reviewed by Smith and Sturmey (2013). The conversion of glucose to lactate is a rapid method of generating ATP, but it is rather inefficient at producing cellular energy. Consequently, the high levels of aerobic glycolysis may not be intended solely to respond to the increasing energy requirements of the blastocyst. Other reasons could be the provision of precursors for biosynthetic processes (e.g., synthesis of proteins, lipids, complex sugars, and moieties for nucleic acid synthesis as well as NADPH from metabolizing glucose though the pentose phosphate pathway (Lewis & Sturmey, 2015) and the adaptation of the blastocyst to the hypoxic environment during implantation (Leese, 1995). One intriguing idea to explain the rise in glycolysis is the increase in production of lactate, which when excreted will cause a local fall in pH. It was postulated by Gardner that this might be important in facilitating invasive implantation (Gardner, 2015).

4.4 What Are the Major Sources of Stress for the Embryo?

4.4.1 In Vitro vs. In Vivo

From fertilization to implantation in vivo, the embryo is exposed to dynamic conditions of pH, nutrient availability, and oxygen levels through the female genital tract. These physiological conditions differ markedly compared to the environment in vitro, which compromise their homeostasis and elicit stress responses. As in vivo studies in human are largely impractical, animal models have provided valuable knowledge about the different regulation of metabolism occurring between in vivo vs. in vitro embryos. The mouse is considered an appropriate animal model to study this comparison due to the ease and speed of collecting in vivo-derived embryos. Thus, it has been reported that the glycolytic rates of in vitro-derived blastocysts are higher than those of in vivo blastocysts and this is associated with decreased implantation and viability after transfer (Gardner & Leese, 1990; Lane & Gardner, 1996; 1998). Exposing in vivo-developed mice blastocysts to in vitro culture conditions induces metabolic adaptation in just 3 hours. Such effects are milder when in vivo-derived blastocysts are cultured in the presence of amino acids and vitamins, underlining the importance of culture media composition for correct metabolic status (Lane & Gardner, 1998). The impact of in vitro culture on metabolism can also be seen in cattle embryos, which exhibit reduced glucose oxidation – and therefore higher glycolysis, in agreement with data from mice – and higher amino acid turnover compared to their in vivo-derived counterparts (Thompson, 1997; Sturmey et al., 2010). The extent of this impact in embryo development is time-dependent: the longer the exposure to in vitro conditions, the higher the impact (Merton et al., 2003). In vitro culture also induces changes in gene expression related to lipid metabolism and oxidative stress, as shown when in vitro vs. in vivo generated cattle or porcine blastocysts were compared (Bauer et al., 2010; Gad et al., 2012). Moreover, DNA methylation patterns are also affected by in vitro conditions, leading to the transmission of hypomethylated marks on imprinted genes in in vivo-derived cattle blastocysts exposed to in vitro culture before the EGA (Salilew-Wondim et al., 2018).

4.5 How Are Stress and Metabolism Linked?

Gamete and embryo manipulation in vitro cause cellular stress, which is linked to altered gene expression patterns. This occurs through stress pathways, such as altered metabolic status, in response to environmental perturbations (Leese et al., 1998; Thompson et al., 2002). Whether there are particularly sensitive windows of development remains unclear. However, one view is that the embryo is more sensitive to environmental stress before EGA occurs (Brison et al., 2014).

Intracellular pH undoubtedly affects metabolic activity by altering the activity of different enzymes and disruption of specific molecular pathways, including glycolytic and oxidative metabolism (Edwards et al., 1998b; Lane & Gardner, 2000). Human embryos have the ability to buffer their own intracellular pH to a certain extent (Phillips et al., 2000). In mice, buffering capacity is stronger from compaction and blastocyst formation, when the number of cell–cell junctions increases (Edwards et al., 1998a). This plasticity makes sense, considering the physiological conditions as the embryo is successively exposed to change from alkaline pH in the fallopian tube (pH 7.1–8.4) to a more acidic pH (pH 7.3–7.9) in the uterine endometrium (Ng et al., 2018). However, this plasticity can be modified by extracellular pH in culture conditions; slight variations in the extracellular pH during embryo manipulation in mice led to developmental and genetic disorders (Koustas & Sjoblom, 2011). The aspects of pH in the culture environment have been reviewed in detail in Swain, 2010 and Swain, 2012. Concomitant with pH is the effect of temperature in culture systems, as any variation is reflected by a change in pH (Wale & Gardner, 2016). This is usually solved by using buffering systems (e.g., bicarbonate/carbon dioxide).

The concentration of ambient oxygen can further impact embryo development and reproductive outcome. In all mammalian species including humans, atmospheric oxygen levels (20%) have proved inferior compared to low oxygen levels (5%) at supporting both cleavage and post-compaction stages of development (Thompson et al., 1990; Batt et al., 1991; Catt & Henman, 2000; Kovacic & Vlaisavljevic, 2008; Kovacic et al., 2010; Wale & Gardner, 2010; Bontekoe et al., 2012; Zaninovic et al., 2013). This is unsurprising, given that the physiological oxygen levels in the mammalian oviduct range from 5 to 8.7% (Fischer & Bavister, 1993). Indeed, oxygen levels in the female reproductive tract drop from 5 to 7% in the fallopian tube to around 2% in the uterus, where implantation occurs (Fischer & Bavister, 1993). Based on that, it has been recently suggested that in vitro culture systems with ultra-low levels of oxygen (2%) from the blastocyst stage were advantageous for embryo development (Morin et al., 2017; Kaser et al., 2018). However, other studies did not find any effect after sequential in vitro culture from low to ultra-low oxygen levels (De Munck et al., 2019).

The metabolism of oxygen is important for embryo development, but it can be a source of oxidative stress via the production of reactive oxygen species (ROS). Low levels of ROS, which are produced as a result of redox reactions and oxidative phosphorylation, are needed to ensure correct signaling pathways in physiological conditions (Hancock et al., 2001). However, rising levels of ROS can cause ATP depletion, mitochondrial damage, DNA damage, and alterations of cell constituents, such as lipids and proteins (Guerin et al., 2001), as well as developmental arrest (Balaban et al., 2005; Favetta et al., 2007). Although the optimal metabolic conditions to ensure a proper oxidative balance have not been established, the inclusion of compounds such as metal chelators, thioredoxin, and certain vitamins can help regulate embryonic ROS production (Guerin et al., 2001). Results from experiments in mice suggest that the addition of antioxidants to the culture media may be beneficial (Truong et al., 2016; Truong & Gardner, 2017).

Ammonium, which is toxic for mammalian embryos, is spontaneously built up from amino acid deamination at 37°C. Under stress, embryos release increased amounts of ammonium and lactate to the culture medium, modifying the intracellular pH, and unbalancing the glycolytic activity in order to restore homeostasis (Lane & Gardner, 2000; Lane & Gardner, 2003; Dagilgan et al., 2015). High levels of ammonium in culture medium can result in the differential expression of genes involved in metabolism, cell communication, and development, among others (Gardner et al., 2013). Of note, it has been reported that ammonium levels can accumulate in IVF culture medium, both following prolonged storage and also at 37°C when supplemented with glutamine and proteins (Kleijkers et al., 2016). This is enhanced by culture at atmospheric oxygen levels (Wale & Gardner, 2013). Importantly, both oxygen and ammonium alter the overall amino acid metabolism in an independent manner, high oxygen being the most detrimental (Orsi & Leese, 2004b; Wale & Gardner, 2013).

4.6 Can We Use Metabolism to Minimize Stress?

Each of the stress-derived effects described above relies on the disturbance of embryo metabolic homeostasis. These effects are likely to persist throughout the post-natal life and subsequent generations by changing transcriptional expression and epigenetic patterns according to the Developmental Origins of Health and Disease (DOHaD) hypothesis (Barker, 2007; Reid et al., 2017).

Stress-related effects in in vitro culture systems clearly influence the outcome of in vitro embryo technologies, but is it possible to reverse those effects? The idea of manipulating metabolism in vitro to improve IVF outcomes is tempting and seems feasible, especially given that the metabolic profile of embryos can be modified comparatively simply. For example, studies in mice have shown that maternal low protein diet during the preimplantation period induce metabolic changes in the maternal serum and uterine secretions, showing reduced insulin and amino acids and increased glucose levels in serum, as well as reduced amino acid availability in the uterine fluid. Those changes were concomitant with abnormal blastocyst growth and metabolic signaling, which the authors interpreted as compensatory responses to the environmental challenges sensed by the embryo (Eckert et al., 2012). The transfer of blastocysts cultured in insulin and amino acid-depleted media in a follow-up study resulted in higher weight (both at birth and early postnatal life), increased blood pressure in males, and decreased heart to body weight ratio in females compared to controls (Velazquez et al., 2018). In another example, it was recently reported that the administration of a mitochondrial targeted antioxidant can rescue the developmental competence and quality of cattle embryos exposed to lipotoxicity and oxidative stress during oocyte maturation (Marei et al., 2019).

In mice, it has been reported that advanced maternal age induces altered programming in blastocysts leading to abnormal postnatal cardiometabolic profiles, i.e., body weight, blood pressure, and glucose metabolism (Velazquez et al., 2016). Supplementation of the culture medium with dichloroacetic acid, a stimulator of pyruvate dehydrogenase, boosted the mitochondrial activity and improved the development of embryos derived from aged mice (McPherson et al., 2014). Whether such responses would be apparent in human embryos is unknown, but negative effects of maternal ageing include increased aneuploidy rates (Capalbo et al., 2017; Shi et al., 2019), preterm birth (Kenny et al., 2013) and low birth weight (Fall et al., 2015). The idea of adapting the composition of culture medium to influence metabolism with the intention of minimizing negative responses to stress is therefore a fascinating avenue for future study. However, like any new

Glucose	Low/negligible consumption	Low/negligible consumption	Low/negligible consumption	Rising consumption	High consumption
Lactate	Modest production	Modest Production	Modest Production	Rising production	High Production
Pyruvate	High consumption	High consumption	High consumption	Falling consumption	Low consumption
EAA	Turned over	Turned over	Turned over	Turned over	Turned over
NEAA	Turned over	Turned over	Turned over	Turned over	Turned over
OCR	Low	Low	Low	Rising	High
Glycolysis	Low	Low	Low	Low	High
OXPHOS	Modest	Modest	Modest	Modest	High

Figure 4.2 Summary 'heatmap' of embryo metabolism. Increasing color intensity indicates increased activity, with red indicating substrate depletion and green indicating release. Blue represents 'activity'. For color version of this figure. Please refer color plate section.

advances in reproductive medicine, any research into this area must be fully supported by well conducted randomized control trials and subsequent follow-up before made widely available to patients.

4.7 Summary, Conclusion, and Future Prospects

In summary, the embryo undergoes dynamic changes during preimplantation development showing concordant utilization patterns of substrates such as glucose, lactate, pyruvate, amino acids, and fatty acids – summarized in Figure 4.2. These nutrients play important roles beyond energy production. The embryo is responsive to the external environment and this response is driven by its metabolic activity, which ultimately also determines its genetic status. Metabolic profiling may have some utility as a non-invasive approach to give us a snapshot of embryo physiology. However, there are some methodological limitations hampering translation of metabolic studies. In the way it has been done so far, measuring metabolism does not directly focus on specific pathways or the flux of metabolites across them, but only the end products of metabolism at specific and static time points. Furthermore, all current knowledge about human embryos is derived from either in vitro studies or animal studies. Many aspects of the physio-logical preimplantation environment remain to be discovered and could allow us to improve on current IVF outcomes; an example of this is the fact that adding low doses of oviduct and uterine fluid to the culture medium improves embryo quality and development in cattle (Hamdi et al., 2018). Apart from the variety of molecules mentioned in this chapter which are present in the oviduct and the uterus, other components such as miRNA and extracellular vesicles remain comparatively unexplored; the effects of these compounds in embryo development are unknown.

Emerging data suggest that IVF might affect the health of the offspring and in vitro culture systems are in some aspects being questioned (Sunde et al., 2016). Over 8 million babies have been born from IVF worldwide (De Geyter et al., 2018). These data highlight the importance of developing controlled in vitro culture systems in order to ensure the safety of IVF children. Culture media, pH, temperature, and oxygen levels are some of the factors that should be carefully considered. In conclusion, culture systems should fulfil the energy demands of the embryo but must also balance their metabolic homeostasis. Optimization of media formulations must be based on evidence, and the application of any change in their composition as well as any new technology to the IVF clinical context must be carefully evaluated (Harper et al., 2012).

References

Aguilar J, Reyley M. The uterine tubal fluid: secretion, composition and biological effects. *Anim Reprod.* 2005;2:91–105.

Balaban RS, Nemoto S, Finkel T. Mitochondria, oxidants, and aging. *Cell.* 2005;120:483–495.

Barker DJ. The origins of the developmental origins theory. *J Intern Med.* 2007;261:412–417.

Batt PA, Gardner DK, Cameron AW. Oxygen concentration and protein source affect the development of preimplantation goat embryos in vitro. *Reprod Fertil Dev.* 1991;3:601–607.

Bauer BK, Isom SC, Spate LD, et al. Transcriptional profiling by deep sequencing identifies differences in mRNA transcript abundance in in vivo-derived versus in vitro-cultured porcine blastocyst stage embryos. *Biol Reprod.* 2010;83:791–798.

Baumann CG, Morris DG, Sreenan JM, Leese HJ. The quiet embryo hypothesis: molecular characteristics favoring viability. *Mol Reprod Dev.* 2007;74:1345–1353.

Bontekoe S, Mantikou E, van Wely M, Seshadri S, Repping S, Mastenbroek S. Low oxygen concentrations for embryo culture in assisted reproductive technologies. *Cochrane Database Syst Rev.* 2012; (7), CD008950.

Bradley J, Pope I, Masia F, et al. Quantitative imaging of lipids in live mouse oocytes and early embryos using CARS microscopy. *Development.* 2016;143:2238–2247.

Brison DR, Houghton FD, Falconer D, et al. Identification of viable embryos in IVF by non-invasive measurement of amino acid turnover. *Hum Reprod.* 2004;19:2319–2324.

Brison DR, Sturmey RG, Leese HJ. Metabolic heterogeneity during preimplantation development: the missing link? *Hum Reprod Update.* 2014;20:632–640.

Cagnone G, Sirar, A. The embryonic stress response to in vitro culture: insight from genomic analysis. *Reproduction.* 2016;152:R247–R261.

Capalbo A, Hoffmann ER, Cimadomo D, Ubaldi FM, Rienzi L. Human female meiosis revised: new insights into the mechanisms of chromosome segregation and aneuploidies from advanced genomics and time-lapse imaging. *Hum Reprod Update.* 2017;23:706–722.

Castillo CM, Horne G, Fitzgerald CT, et al. The impact of IVF on birthweight from 1991 to 2015: a cross-sectional study. *Hum Reprod.* 2019;34:920–931.

Catt JW, Henman M. Toxic effects of oxygen on human embryo development. *Hum Reprod.* 2000;15 (Suppl 2):199–206.

Chen PR, Redel BK, Spate LD, Ji T, Salazar SR, Prather RS. Glutamine supplementation enhances development of in vitro-produced porcine embryos and increases leucine consumption from the medium. *Biol Reprod.* 2018;99:938–948.

Cheong Y, Boomsma C, Heijnen C, Macklon N. Uterine secretomics: a window on the maternal-embryo interface. *Fertil Steril.* 2013;99:1093–1099.

Coticchio G, Lagalla C, Sturmey R, Pennetta F, Borini A. The enigmatic morula: mechanisms of development, cell fate determination, self-correction and implications for ART. *Hum Reprod Update.* 2019;25:422–438.

Coull G, Speake B, Staines M, Broadbent P, McEvoy T. Lipid and fatty acid composition of zona-intact sheep oocytes. *Theriogenology.* 1998;49:179.

Crosby IM, Gandolfi F, Moor RM. Control of protein synthesis during early cleavage of sheep embryos. *J Reprod Fertil.* 1988;82:769–775.

Dagilgan S, Dundar-Yenilmez E, Tuli A, Urunsak IF, Erdogan S. Evaluation of intracellular pH regulation and alkalosis defense mechanisms in preimplantation embryos. *Theriogenology.* 2015;83:1075–1084.

Dawson KM, Baltz JM. Organic osmolytes and embryos: substrates of the Gly and beta transport systems protect mouse zygotes against the effects of raised osmolarity. *Biol Reprod.* 1997;56:1550–1558.

De Geyter C, Calhaz-Jorge C, Kupka MS, et al. ART in Europe, 2014: results generated from European registries by ESHRE: The European IVF-monitoring Consortium (EIM) for the European Society of Human Reproduction and Embryology (ESHRE). *Hum Reprod.* 2018;33:1586–1601.

De Munck N, Janssens R, Segers I, Tournaye H, Van de Velde H, Verheyen G. Influence of ultra-low oxygen (2%) tension on in-vitro human embryo development. *Hum Reprod.* 2019;34:228–234.

Devreker F, Winston RM, Hardy K. Glutamine improves human preimplantation development in vitro. *Fertil Steril.* 1998;69;293–299.

Eckert JJ, Houghton FD, Hawkhead JA, et al. Human embryos developing in vitro are susceptible to impaired epithelial junction biogenesis correlating with abnormal metabolic activity. *Hum Reprod.* 2007;22:2214–2224.

Eckert JJ, Porter R, Watkins AJ, et al. Metabolic induction and early responses of mouse blastocyst developmental programming following maternal low protein diet affecting life-long health. *PLoS One.* 2012;7:e52791.

Edwards LJ, Williams DA, Gardner DK. Intracellular pH of the mouse preimplantation embryo: amino acids act as buffers of intracellular pH. *Hum Reprod.* 1998a;13:3441–3448.

Intracellular pH of the preimplantation mouse embryo: effects of extracellular pH and weak acids. *Mol Reprod Dev.* 1998b;50:434–442.

Epstein CJ, Smith SA. Amino acid uptake and protein synthesis in preimplanatation mouse embryos. *Dev Biol.* 1973;33:171–184.

Fall CH, Sachdev HS, Osmond C, et al. Association between maternal age at childbirth and child and adult outcomes in the offspring: a prospective study in five low-income and middle-income countries (COHORTS collaboration). *Lancet Glob Health.* 2015;3:e366–377.

Favetta LA, St John EJ, King WA, Betts DH. High levels of p66shc and intracellular ROS in permanently arrested early embryos. *Free Radic Biol Med.* 2007;42:1201–1210.

Ferguson EM, Leese HJ. Triglyceride content of bovine oocytes and early embryos. *J Reprod Fertil.* 1999;116:373–378.

Fernandez-Gonzalez R, Moreira P, Bilbao A, et al. Long-term effect of in vitro culture of mouse embryos with serum on mRNA expression of imprinting genes, development, and behavior. *Proc Natl Acad Sci U S A.* 2004;101:5880–5885.

Fischer B, Bavister BD. Oxygen tension in the oviduct and uterus of rhesus monkeys, hamsters and rabbits. *J Reprod Fertil.* 1993;99:673–679.

Gad A, Hoelker M, Besenfelder U, et al. Molecular mechanisms and pathways involved in bovine embryonic genome activation and their regulation by alternative in vivo and in vitro culture conditions. *Biol Reprod.* 2012;87:100.

Gardner DK. Changes in requirements and utilization of nutrients during mammalian preimplantation embryo development and their significance in embryo culture. *Theriogenology.* 1998;49; 83–102.

Metabolism of the viable embryo. In: Gardner DK, Sakkas D, Seli E, Wells D, ed. *Emerging Technologies for the Assessment and Diagnosis of Gametes and Embryos.* New York: Springer; 2013:211–223.

Lactate production by the mammalian blastocyst: manipulating the microenvironment for uterine implantation and invasion? *Bioessays.* 2015;37:364–371.

Gardner DK, Hamilton R, McCallie B, Schoolcraft WB, Katz-Jaffe MG. Human and mouse embryonic development, metabolism and gene expression are altered by an ammonium gradient in vitro. *Reproduction.* 2013;146:49–61.

Gardner DK, Lane M, Calderon I, Leeton J. Environment of the preimplantation human embryo in vivo: metabolite analysis of oviduct and uterine fluids and metabolism of cumulus cells. *Fertil Steril.* 1996;65:349–353.

Gardner DK, Leese HJ. Concentrations of nutrients in mouse oviduct fluid and their effects on embryo development and metabolism in vitro. *J Reprod Fertil.* 1990;88:361–368.

Gardner DK, Wale P, Collins R, Lane M. Glucose consumption of single post-compaction human embryos is predictive of embryo sex and live birth outcome. *Hum Reprod.* 2011;26:1981–1986.

Gonzalez IM, Martin PM, Burdsal C, et al. Leucine and arginine regulate trophoblast motility through mTOR-dependent and independent pathways in the preimplantation mouse embryo. *Dev Biol.* 2012;361:286–300.

Goto K, Kumasako Y, Koike M, et al. Prediction of the in vitro developmental competence of early-cleavage-stage human embryos with time-lapse imaging and oxygen consumption rate measurement. *Reprod Med Biol.* 2018;17:289–296.

Guerif F, McKeegan P, Leese HJ, Sturmey RG. A simple approach for COnsumption and RElease (CORE) analysis of metabolic activity in single mammalian embryos. *PLoS One.* 2013;8: e67834.

Guerin P, El Mouatassim S, Menezo Y. Oxidative stress and protection against reactive oxygen species in the pre-implantation embryo and its surroundings. *Hum Reprod Update.* 2001;7:175–189.

Haggarty P, Wood M, Ferguson E, et al. Fatty acid metabolism in human preimplantation embryos. *Hum Reprod.* 2006;21:766–773.

Hamdi M, Lopera-Vasquez R, Maillo V, et al. Bovine oviductal and uterine fluid support in vitro embryo development. *Reprod Fertil Dev.* 2018;30:935–945.

Hancock JT, Desikan R, Neill SJ. Role of reactive oxygen species in cell signalling pathways. *Biochem Soc Trans.* 2001;29:345–350.

Harper J, Magli MC, Lundin K, Barratt CL, Brison D. When and how should new technology be introduced into the IVF laboratory? *Hum Reprod.* 2012;27:303–313.

Houghton FD, Hawkhead JA, Humpherson PG, et al. Non-invasive amino acid turnover predicts human embryo developmental capacity. *Hum Reprod.* 2002;17:999–1005.

Houghton FD, Humpherson PG, Hawkhead JA, Hall CJ, Leese HJ. Na$^+$, K$^+$, ATPase activity in the human and bovine preimplantation embryo. *Dev Bio.* 2003;263:360–366.

Houghton FD, Thompson JG, Kennedy CJ, Leese HJ. Oxygen consumption and energy metabolism of the early mouse embryo. *Mol Reprod Dev.* 1996;44:476–485.

Humpherson PG, Leese HJ, Sturmey RG. Amino acid metabolism of the porcine blastocyst. *Theriogenology.* 2005;64:1852–1866.

Kaser DJ, Bogale B, Sarda V, Farland LV, Williams PL, Racowsky C. Randomized controlled trial of low (5%) versus ultralow (2%) oxygen for extended culture using bipronucleate and tripronucleate human preimplantation embryos. *Fertil Steril*. 2018;109:1030–1037 e2.

Kenny LC, Lavender T, McNamee R, O'Neill SM, Mills T, Khashan AS. Advanced maternal age and adverse pregnancy outcome: evidence from a large contemporary cohort. *PLoS One*. 2013;8:e56583.

Kermack AJ, Finn-Sell S, Cheong YC, et al. Amino acid composition of human uterine fluid: association with age, lifestyle and gynaecological pathology. *Hum Reprod*. 2015; 30:917–924.

Kleijkers SH, van Montfoort AP, Bekers O, et al. Ammonium accumulation in commercially available embryo culture media and protein supplements during storage at 2–8 degrees C and during incubation at 37 degrees C. *Hum Reprod*. 2016; 31:1192–1199.

Koustas G, Sjoblom C. Epigenetic consequences of pH stress in mouse embryos. *Hum Reprod*. 2011;26(suppl_1):i78.

Kovacic B, Sajko MC, Vlaisavljevic V. A prospective, randomized trial on the effect of atmospheric versus reduced oxygen concentration on the outcome of intracytoplasmic sperm injection cycles. *Fertil Steri*. 2010;94:511–519.

Kovacic B, Vlaisavljevic V. Influence of atmospheric versus reduced oxygen concentration on development of human blastocysts in vitro: a prospective study on sibling oocytes. *Reprod Biomed Online*. 2008;17:229–236.

Lane M, Gardner DK. Selection of viable mouse blastocysts prior to transfer using a metabolic criterion. *Hum Reprod*. 1996;11:1975–1978.

Amino acids and vitamins prevent culture-induced metabolic perturbations and associated loss of viability of mouse blastocysts. *Hum Reprod*. 1998;13:991–997.

Regulation of ionic homeostasis by mammalian embryos. *Semin Reprod Med*. 2000;18:195–204.

Ammonium induces aberrant blastocyst differentiation, metabolism, pH regulation, gene expression and subsequently alters fetal development in the mouse. *Biol Reprod*. 2003;69:1109–1117.

Mitochondrial malate-aspartate shuttle regulates mouse embryo nutrient consumption. *J Biol Chem*. 2005a;280:18361–18367.

Understanding cellular disruptions during early embryo development that perturb viability and fetal development. *Reprod Fertil Dev*. 2005b;17: 371–378.

Leese HJ. The formation and function of oviduct fluid. *J Reprod Fertil*. 1988;82:843–856.

Metabolic control during preimplantation mammalian development. *Hum Reprod Update*. 1995;1:63–72.

Quiet please, do not disturb: a hypothesis of embryo metabolism and viability. *Bioessays*. 2002;24:845–849.

Metabolism of the preimplantation embryo: 40 years on. *Reproduction*. 2012;143:417–427.

Leese HJ, Barton AM. Pyruvate and glucose uptake by mouse ova and preimplantation embryos. *J Reprod Fertil*. 1984;72:9–13.

Production of pyruvate by isolated mouse cumulus cells. *J Exp Zool*. 1985;234:231–236.

Leese HJ, Baumann CG, Brison DR, McEvoy TG, Sturmey RG. Metabolism of the viable mammalian embryo: quietness revisited. *Mol Hum Reprod*. 2008a;14:667–672.

Leese HJ, Conaghan J, Martin KL, Hardy K. Early human embryo metabolism. *Bioessays*. 1993;15:259–264.

Leese HJ, Donnay I, Thompson JG. Human assisted conception: a cautionary tale. Lessons from domestic animals. *Hum Reprod*. 1998;13(Suppl 4):184–202.

Leese HJ, Guerif F, Allgar V, Brison DR, Lundin K, Sturmey RG. Biological optimization, the Goldilocks principle, and how much is lagom in the preimplantation embryo. *Mol Reprod Dev*. 2016;83:748–754.

Leese HJ, Hugentobler SA, Gray SM, et al. Female reproductive tract fluids: composition, mechanism of formation and potential role in the developmental origins of health and disease. *Reprod Fertil Dev*. 2008b;20:1–8.

Leese HJ, Sathyapalan T, Allgar V, Brison DR, Sturmey R. Going to extremes: the Goldilocks/Lagom principle and data distribution. *BMJ Open*. 2019;9:e027767.

Leese HJ, Sturmey RG, Baumann CG, McEvoy TG. Embryo viability and metabolism: obeying the quiet rules. *Hum Reprod*. 2007;22:3047–3050.

Leroy JL, Genicot G, Donnay I, Van Soom, A. Evaluation of the lipid content in bovine oocytes and embryos with nile red: a practical approach. *Reprod Domest Anim*. 2005;40:76–87.

Lewis N, Sturmey RG. Embryo metabolism: what does it really mean? *Anim. Reprod*. 12;2015:521–528.

Marei WFA, Van den Bosch L, Pintelon I, Mohey-Elsaeed O, Bols PEJ, Leroy J. Mitochondria-targeted therapy rescues development and quality of embryos derived from oocytes matured under oxidative stress conditions: a bovine in vitro model. *Hum Reprod*. 2019;34:1984–1998.

Matorras R, Ruiz JI, Mendoza R, Ruiz N, Sanjurjo P, Rodriguez-Escudero FJ. Fatty acid composition of fertilization-failed human oocytes. *Hum Reprod.* 1998;13:2227–2230.

McEvoy TG, Coull GD, Broadbent PJ, Hutchinson JS, Speake BK. Fatty acid composition of lipids in immature cattle, pig and sheep oocytes with intact zona pellucida. *J Reprod Fertil.* 2000;118:163–170.

McPherson NO, Zander-Fox D, Lane M. Stimulation of mitochondrial embryo metabolism by dichloroacetic acid in an aged mouse model improves embryo development and viability. *Fertil Steril.* 2014;101:1458–1466.

Merton JS, de Roos AP, Mullaart E, et al. Factors affecting oocyte quality and quantity in commercial application of embryo technologies in the cattle breeding industry. *Theriogenology.* 2003;59:651–674.

Mitchell M, Cashman KS, Gardner DK, Thompson JG, Lane M. Disruption of mitochondrial malate-aspartate shuttle activity in mouse blastocysts impairs viability and fetal growth. *Biol Reprod.* 2009;80:295–301.

Morin SJ, Kaser DJ, Juneau CR, et al. The LO2 trial, phase 1: a paired randomized controlled trial (RCT) comparing blastulation rate in ultra-low (2%) vs. low (5%) oxygen in extended culture. *Fertil Steril* 2017;108(3 suppl):e58–59.

Nagaraj R, Sharpley MS, Chi F, et al. Nuclear localization of mitochondrial TCA cycle enzymes as a critical step in mammalian zygotic genome activation. *Cell.* 2017;168:210–223 e11.

Ng KYB, Mingels R, Morgan H, Macklon N, Cheong Y. In vivo oxygen, temperature and pH dynamics in the female reproductive tract and their importance in human conception: a systematic review. *Hum Reprod Update.* 2018;24:15–34.

Orsi NM, Leese HJ. Amino acid metabolism of preimplantation bovine embryos cultured with bovine serum albumin or polyvinyl alcohol. *Theriogenology,* 2004a;61:561–572.

Ammonium exposure and pyruvate affect the amino acid metabolism of bovine blastocysts in vitro. *Reproduction.* 2004b;127:131–140.

Phillips KP, Leveille MC, Claman P, Baltz JM. Intracellular pH regulation in human preimplantation embryos. *Hum Reprod.* 2000;15:896–904.

Picton HM, Elder K, Houghton FD, et al. Association between amino acid turnover and chromosome aneuploidy during human preimplantation embryo development in vitro. *Mol Hum Reprod.* 2010;16:557–569.

Redel BK, Brown AN, Spate LD, Whitworth KM, Green JA, Prather RS. Glycolysis in preimplantation development is partially controlled by the Warburg effect. *Mol Reprod Dev.* 2012;79:262–271.

Reid MA, Dai Z, Locasale JW. The impact of cellular metabolism on chromatin dynamics and epigenetics. *Nat Cell Biol.* 2017;19:1298–1306.

Rezk Y, Huff C, Rizk B. Effect of glutamine on preimplantation mouse embryo development in vitro. *Am J Obstet Gynecol.* 2004;190:1450–1454.

Salilew-Wondim D, Saeed-Zidane M, Hoelker M, et al. Genome-wide DNA methylation patterns of bovine blastocysts derived from in vivo embryos subjected to in vitro culture before, during or after embryonic genome activation. *BMC Genomics.* 2018;19:424.

Shi Y, Ma J, Xue Y, Wang J, Yu B, Wang T. The assessment of combined karyotype analysis and chromosomal microarray in pregnant women of advanced maternal age: a multicenter study. *Ann Transl Med.* 2019;7:318.

Smith DG, Sturmey RG. Parallels between embryo and cancer cell metabolism. *Biochem Soc Trans.* 2013;41:664–669.

Steeves TE, Gardner DK. Temporal and differential effects of amino acids on bovine embryo development in culture. *Biol Reprod.* 1999;61:731–740.

Stokes PJ, Hawkhead JA, Fawthrop RK, et al. Metabolism of human embryos following cryopreservation: implications for the safety and selection of embryos for transfer in clinical IVF. *Hum Reprod.* 2007;22:829–835.

Sturmey RG, Bermejo-Alvarez P, Gutierrez-Adan A, Rizos D, Leese HJ, Lonergan P. Amino acid metabolism of bovine blastocysts: a biomarker of sex and viability. *Mol Reprod Dev.* 2010;77:285–296.

Sturmey RG, Brison DR, Leese HJ. Symposium: innovative techniques in human embryo viability assessment. Assessing embryo viability by measurement of amino acid turnover. *Reprod Biomed Online.* 2008;17:486–496.

Sturmey RG, Hawkhead JA, Barker EA, Leese HJ. DNA damage and metabolic activity in the preimplantation embryo. *Hum Reprod.* 2009;24:81–91.

Sturmey RG, Leese HJ. Energy metabolism in pig oocytes and early embryos. *Reproduction.* 2003;126:197–204.

Sturmey RG, O'Toole PJ, Leese HJ. Fluorescence resonance energy transfer analysis of mitochondrial: lipid association in the porcine oocyte. *Reproduction.* 2006;132:829–837.

Sudano MJ, Paschoal DM, Rascado Tda S, et al. Lipid content and apoptosis of in vitro-produced bovine embryos as determinants of susceptibility to vitrification. *Theriogenology.* 2011;75:1211–1220.

Summers MC, Biggers JD. Chemically defined media and the culture of mammalian preimplantation embryos: historical perspective and current issues. *Hum Reprod Update.* 2003;9:557–582.

Sunde A, Brison D, Dumoulin J, et al. Time to take human embryo culture seriously. *Hum Reprod.* 2016;31:2174–2182.

Suzuki C, Yoshioka K, Sakatani M, Takahashi M. Glutamine and hypotaurine improves intracellular oxidative status and in vitro development of porcine preimplantation embryos. *Zygote.* 2007;15:317–324.

Swain JE. Optimizing the culture environment in the IVF laboratory: impact of pH and buffer capacity on gamete and embryo quality. *Reprod Biomed Online.* 2010;21:6–16.

Is there an optimal pH for culture media used in clinical IVF? *Hum Reprod Update.* 2012;18:333–339.

Tatsumi T, Takayama K, Ishii S et al. Forced lipophagy reveals that lipid droplets are required for early embryonic development in mouse. *Development.* 2018;145: dev161893.

Thompson JG. Comparison between in vivo-derived and in vitro-produced pre-elongation embryos from domestic ruminants. *Reprod Fertil Dev.* 1997;9:341–354.

Thompson JG, Kind KL, Roberts CT, Robertson SA, Robinson JS. Epigenetic risks related to assisted reproductive technologies: short- and long-term consequences for the health of children conceived through assisted reproduction technology: more reason for caution? *Hum Reprod.* 2002;17:2783–2786.

Thompson JG, Partridge RJ, Houghton FD, Cox CI, Leese HJ. Oxygen uptake and carbohydrate metabolism by in vitro derived bovine embryos. *J Reprod Fertil.* 1996;106:299–306.

Thompson JG, Simpson AC, Pugh PA, Donnelly PE, Tervit HR. Effect of oxygen concentration on in-vitro development of preimplantation sheep and cattle embryos. *J Reprod Fertil.* 1990;89:573–578.

Truong T, Gardner DK. Antioxidants improve IVF outcome and subsequent embryo development in the mouse. *Hum Reprod.* 2017;32:2404–2413.

Truong TT, Soh YM, Gardner DK. Antioxidants improve mouse preimplantation embryo development and viability. *Hum Reprod.* 2016;31:1445–1454.

Van Winkle LJ, Tesch JK, Shah A, Campione L. System B0,+ amino acid transport regulates the penetration stage of blastocyst implantation with possible long-term developmental consequences through adulthood. *Hum Reprod Update.* 2006;12:145–157.

Velazquez MA, Sheth B, Smith SJ, Eckert JJ, Osmond C Fleming TP. Insulin and branched-chain amino acid depletion during mouse preimplantation embryo culture programmes body weight gain and raised blood pressure during early postnatal life. *Biochim Biophys Acta Mol Basis Dis.* 2018;1864;590–600.

Velazquez MA, Smith CG, Smyth NR, Osmond C, Fleming TP. Advanced maternal age causes adverse programming of mouse blastocysts leading to altered growth and impaired cardiometabolic health in post-natal life. *Hum Reprod.* 2016;31:1970–1980.

Wale PL, Gardner DK. Time-lapse analysis of mouse embryo development in oxygen gradients. *Reprod Biomed Online.* 2010;21:402–410.

Oxygen affects the ability of mouse blastocysts to regulate ammonium. *Biol Reprod.* 2013;89:75.

The effects of chemical and physical factors on mammalian embryo culture and their importance for the practice of assisted human reproduction. *Hum Reprod Update.* 2016;22:2–22.

Walther TC, Farese RV, Jr. Lipid droplets and cellular lipid metabolism. *Annu Rev Biochem.* 2012;81:687–714.

Warburg O. On the origin of cancer cells. *Science.* 1956;123:309–314.

Zaninovic N, Goldschlag J, Yin H,Ye Z, Clarke R, Rosenwaks Z. Impact of oxygen concentration on embryo development, embryo morphology and morphokinetics. *Fertil Steril.* 2013;100:S240.

Chapter 5

Culture Media and Embryo Culture

Arne Sunde and Roger G. Sturmey

5.1 What the Medium Does

Before considering the basis of embryo culture medium, it is worthwhile reflecting on its function. A detailed overview of embryo metabolism is given in Chapter 4; however, in brief, the embryo must satisfy changing demands for energy by consumption of nutrients from the external milieu (Lewis & Sturmey, 2015). In an in vivo setting, these needs are catered for in a dynamic manner by the secretions of the oviduct; in an in vitro situation, these requirements must be satisfied by the embryo culture medium. In addition to the provision of energy substrates, the medium must also satisfy basic physico-chemical requirements. Primarily, the medium must facilitate buffering of pH in response both to changing environments to which the embryo is exposed and to excretion of metabolic waste products, notably lactic acid, which is released by cells with accompanying protons, causing pH to fall. Moreover, the culture medium must avoid inducing osmotic stress. One of the major consumers of cellular energy is the maintenance of intracellular ion composition, maintained through the action of ion pumps. Providing suitable osmolarity and pH are among the most basic requirements of any embryo culture medium.

5.2 Culture Media: Historical Perspectives

For as long as there have been attempts to grow embryos outside the body, there has been a need for a medium to support this. Landmark studies performed by the pioneers of embryo development, including Wes Whitten, John Biggers, Ralph Brinster, David Whittingham, and Yves Menezo, paved the way for modern embryo culture. To review the entirety of these significant endeavors would be a book in itself; thus, for an authoritative overview of

the early history of the development of embryo culture, the reader is encouraged to read the excellent account by Chronopolou and Harper (2015). However, much of the outstanding work on optimizing embryo culture medium undertaken by the trailblazers was based on well-educated "guesswork"; a degree of empirical trial and error. However, two specific approaches are worthy of a specific mention.

5.2.1 "Synthetic" Oviduct Fluid

In 1972, Tervit and colleagues reported the successful culture of cattle and sheep ova in vitro (Tervit et al., 1972). In this paper, the authors described in detail the composition of a then-novel culture medium, which they named SOF – Synthetic Oviduct Fluid, an appropriate name since it was synthetic (i.e., created in the laboratory) and able to replicate the role of the fluid within the oviduct. Importantly, the composition of SOF was based on data on the composition of the fluid from the sheep oviduct (Restall & Wales, 1966). Using this medium, combined with an oxygen tension of 5%, Tervit and colleagues were able to generate ovine and cattle blastocysts past the so-called "development block" (which we now know to equate to zygotic genome activation), and, following transfer into suitable recipients, generate pregnancies. Indeed, almost 50 years later, SOF remains the definitive medium for the culture of cattle embryos.

The importance of the development of SOF lies not only in findings but the approach: to produce a medium whose composition was based on the fluids of the genital tract. Such an approach was adopted by Pat Quinn and colleagues (Quinn et al., 1985), who developed an embryo culture medium (human tubal fluid, HTF) based on earlier published reports of the composition of fallopian tube fluid (Lippes et al., 1972; Lopata et al., 1976). In what was probably a world first, Quinn and colleagues undertook a randomized comparison of culture media using human embryos and found that the medium based on the reported composition of the fluid from the oviduct better supported embryo development. Interestingly, Quinn et al. were able to elegantly demonstrate that as the concentration of potassium ions within culture medium fell, so did the blastocyst rate, illustrating the importance of optimized ionic composition of medium for successful embryo culture, and the apparent need for a high potassium content – a phenomenon still not adequately explained (Quinn et al., 1985). By modern standards, this was a small study, comprising of 417 human oocytes; however, it does represent the first dedicated, specific human embryo culture medium. HTF remains the basis of many contemporary embryo culture media.

The concept of seeking inspiration from the in vivo environment to inform strategies for the production of human embryo culture medium underpins the second approach to be considered: sequential medium.

5.2.3 Sequential Embryo Culture

The optimal time to transfer an embryo into the recipient has been intensely debated for many years. In general, there are two schools of thought: transfer the cleavage stage embryo on day 2–3 post insemination or transfer on day 5, or later, when the embryo has formed a blastocyst. Early clinical IVF relied largely on transferring embryos at the cleavage stages, due in part to perceived shortcomings in embryo culture medium (Gardner and Lane, 1998). However, from the early 2000s, there has been a shift toward transferring blastocysts, in large part facilitated by improvements in embryo culture. In vivo, the final stages of gamete maturation, fertilization, and early cleavage occur within the fallopian tube. The embryo resides in this environment for approximately 5 days, after which it transits into the uterus, in readiness for implantation. This transit coincides with the formation of the blastocyst. Since embryos are typically transferred into the uterus, it makes a degree of sense to transfer at the stage of development when they would typically enter the uterus – the blastocyst.

During in vivo development, the movement of the embryo from one anatomical structure to a second may logically be interpreted as a change in environment: one environment for fertilization and cleavage, and a different environment to facilitate blastocyst

development. Indeed, numerous attempts at characterizing the differences in the fluids of the oviduct and uterus have been made. In the late 1960s and through the 1970s, there were a series of attempts to measure the fluid composition of the genital tracts from a range of animals, including sheep (Iritani et al., 1969), rabbit (Iritani et al., 1971), pig (Iritani et al., 1974), and mouse (Borland et al., 1977) to name but a few key reports. Although there were differences between the species, a unifying observation was that the composition of fluid collected from the oviducts differed markedly from that of the uterus. Differences in pH, total protein content, nonprotein nitrogen, energy substrates, and ions were reported, further supporting the notion that the environment that supports the cleavage embryo differed from that where the blastocyst would typically reside. Furthermore, the metabolic activity of blastocysts is notably different to that of the cleavage stage embryo; thus a logical conclusion was to develop culture medium customized for stage-specific needs of early embryos: sequential media.

Perhaps the best known sequential embryo culture system was developed during the 1990s, that is the so-called G-series of culture products (Gardner, 1994; Barnes et al., 1995; Gardner & Lane, 1997). Sequential media were designed to support cleavage development (G1), and compaction and blastocyst development (G2). These media differed in terms of the provision of carbohydrates and amino acids, and were again based on measurements made on the fluids from the oviduct and uterus (Gardner et al., 1996). Trialed initially in mouse embryos (Gardner, 1994), the use of a sequential approach was found to support the development of high quality blastocysts, higher implantation, and better embryo development (Gardner & Lane, 1996).

The medium intended to support the cleavage stages of development is characterized by low glucose and the nonessential amino acids (see Chapter 4 for more details). The rationale behind this was that glucose is utilized in very low amounts through cleavage, with pyruvate and lactate being the preferred energy sources at this stage. Based largely on the work of Chatot et al. (1989), who demonstrated that omission of glucose from embryo culture medium was able to support mouse embryo development through the "2-cell block," a viewpoint flourished that glucose was actually inhibitory for cleavage stage embryos. Indeed, Quinn et al. (1985) produced a modified

HTF lacking glucose and phosphate and reported improved embryo development. This modified medium contained EDTA and glutamine. Thus, EDTA was added to further suppress glycolysis and its presence during the cleavage stages of development was shown to improve development of mouse and cattle embryos (Gardner & Lane, 1997).

The medium designed to support blastocyst development (G2) was characterized by the presence of higher glucose and the nonessential and essential amino acids. Furthermore, EDTA was omitted. Considering the accepted picture of embryo metabolism, such a medium would facilitate a rise in glucose depletion and the absence of EDTA will allow glycolysis to occur – characteristic of blastocyst formation.

Although the idea of changing the culture environment to mimic the transition from the fallopian tube to the uterus is reasonable, it is notable that both essential and nonessential amino acids are present in the oviduct fluid of all commonly studied mammalian species (i.e., mice, rabbit, cattle, pig, sheep, and horse) (Aguilar & Reyley, 2005) as well as the human fallopian tube (Tay et al., 1997). Furthermore, embryos consume and release amino acids, whether they are essential or nonessential, throughout the preimplantation period (Brison et al., 2004). Therefore, it seems logical to add all the amino acids and let the embryo decide, considering that the interactions of amino acids with other nutrients are so far unknown (Ménézo et al., 2013).

Importantly, while sequential culture medium makes a degree of logic, there is no conclusive evidence to support the superiority of one culture modality over the other (Biggers et al., 2002; Macklon et al., 2002, Paternot et al., 2010, Summers et al., 2013, Dieamant et al., 2017). So far, there are no randomized controlled trial comparing all the current culture media together, and it is not possible to make conclusions about which one is the best (Chronopoulou & Harper, 2015; Youssef et al., 2015).

5.3 The Components of Embryo Culture Medium

In general terms, modern commercially available embryo culture media varies from relatively simple salt solutions to complex culture media similar to those intended for continuous culture of mammalian cells (Table 5.1, Morbeck et al., 2014a; Tarahomi et al., 2019).

5.3.1 Protein Supplements

In the early days of embryo culture, the medium in which embryos were grown contained undefined biological supplements, such as egg white (Hammond, 1949), or was even composed entirely of plasma (rabbit embryos: Lewis and Gregory, 1929). Indeed, the medium used by Steptoe and Edwards for the first successful IVF contained patient serum (Steptoe and Edwards, 1978). However, a key observation was reported in 1984 by Menezo and colleagues (Menezo et al., 1984) who compared medium supplemented with human cord serum or 1% human serum albumin (HSA) and observed no difference in ongoing pregnancy rates. This led to the conclusion that serum was not necessary for human embryo development. This was an especially prescient observation, given the later reports that linked the inclusion of serum in animal embryo culture medium to imprinting defects and in utero overgrowth – the so-called large offspring syndrome (Young et al., 1998; Sinclair et al., 2000). Nonetheless, there remains the requirement for the inclusion of a macromolecule source, satisfied largely through the inclusion of protein supplements.

Protein supplements, such as human serum albumin (HSA) and serum substitute supplement (SSS), are extracted from human blood; thus the chemical composition varies between batches and manufacturers (Morbeck et al., 2014b). These extracts are not manufactured *specifically* to be used for embryo culture but rather for in vivo clinical use. It is therefore a challenge for manufacturers to source batches of HSA or SSS. A chemical analysis of different culture media revealed the presence of a number of bioactive substances that are not declared on the label or in the product insert (Dyrlund et al., 2014). The origin of these bioactive substances is most likely the protein supplement that was added to the culture media. One study has found that culturing embryos in media containing different protein supplements resulted in a difference in the birthweight of the offspring suggesting that the source of protein supplement is not trivial (Zhu et al., 2014). Even more startlingly, most preparations contain stabilizers such as octanoic acid that is shown to inhibit growth of embryos (Fredrickson et al., 2015). Thus, the inclusion of protein supplements presents somewhat of a paradox: to date their inclusion remains a necessity for viable clinical embryo production, yet the inclusion of chemically undefined products offers a route for embryos to be exposed to unexpected compounds.

Table 5.1 Composition of two very different commercially available culture media. One with few ingredients and based on simple salt solutions, such as EBSS, and the other a very complex culture medium similar to culture intended for continuous culture of mammalian cells. Human serum albumin is added to both media

Medium based on simple salt solutions	Complex embryo culture medium based on media used for continuous culture of mammalian cells						
$CaCl_2$	$(NH4)_6MO_7O_{24} \cdot 4H_2O$	D-glucose	L-arginine Cl	L-methionine	$MnSO_4$	NH_4VO_3	Aurintricarboxylic acid
$MgSO_4 \cdot 7H_2O$	Acetic acid	Ethanolamine	L-asparagin H_2O	L-phenylalanine	$MnSO_4 \cdot H_2O$	$Ni(NO_3)_2 \cdot 6H_2O$	Fe(II)EDTA
KCl	$CaCl_2$	Ethanol	L-Aspartate	L-Proline	Na pyruvate	Nicotinamide	EDTA-Na_2
NaCl	Cholesterol	$FeSO_4 \cdot 7H_2O$	L-Cys Cl H_2O	L-Serine	Na selenite	Putrecine Cl	HEPES
D-Glucose	Choline Cl	Folic acid	L-Glutamic acid	L-Threonine	Na-Citrate.$2H_2O$	Pyridoxine HCl	Fe(II)EDTA
Citrate.H_2O	Citrate.H_2O	Hypoxanthine	L-Glutamine	L-Tryptophan	Na_2HPO_4	Riboflavin	L-Ala-L-Glut
NaH_2PO_4	Cobalamin	i-Inositol	L-Glycine	L-Tyrosine Na_2	Na_3citrate.$2H_2O$	SeO_2	Pluronic-F-68
$NaHCO_3$	$CoCl_2 \cdot 6H_2O$	KCl	L-Hist Cl.H_2O	L-Valine	NaCl	Thiamine-Cl	PVP 10
Pyruvic acid	$CuSO_4 \cdot 5H_2O$	$KCr(SO_4)_2 \cdot 12H2O$	L-Isoleucine	Linoleic acid	NaH_2PO_4	Thioctic cid	Human recombinant insulin
Penicillin	D-Biotin	KH_2PO_4	L-Leucine	$MgCl_2$	$NaHCO_3$	$ZnSO_4$-7-H2O	Penicillin
Streptomycin	D-Ca pantothenate	L-Alanine	L-Lysine	$MgSO_4 \cdot 7H_2O$	$NH_4Al(SO_4)_2 \cdot 12 H_2O$	Phenol red	Gentamicin

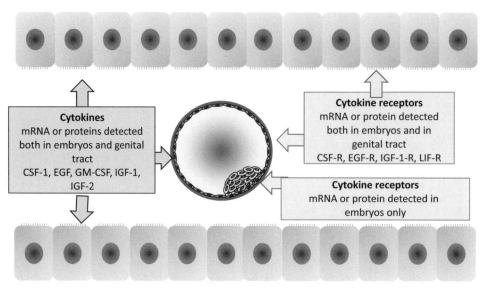

Figure 5.1 Cytokines and cytokine receptors detected in human genital tract and/or in human embryos. Adapted from data published by Wydooghe et al., 2017. For color version of this figure. Please refer color plate section.

Fortunately, significant research in the animal embryo field persists on identifying chemically defined alternatives for embryo culture with some promising results (e.g., Gómez et al., 2020).

Beyond the presence of protein supplements, some culture media contain added hormones and growth factors in addition to the various protein supplements.

5.3.2 Growth Factors and Hormones

The fluid within the genital tract contains a myriad of bioactive proteins and their receptors (Figure 5.1). It is not unreasonable to assume that the concentration of these growth factors in vivo is carefully controlled and may change during the menstrual cycle. Additionally, there is likely a difference between the proximal and distal end of the fallopian tube as well as in the uterus. In vivo, these growth factors may exert their putative effect on gametes, zygotes, and embryos acting both directly and indirectly by modulating the functions of the various cells in the genital tract. However, there is an almost complete absence of data enabling a systematic approach to identify which growth factor(s) to add to embryo culture media and at which concentration. Therefore, most embryo culture media do not contain added growth factors despite the prediction that, in vivo, they play an important role in regulating growth and differentiation of early embryos.

Cytokines are molecules primarily regulating the function of cells involved in the immune response. Several cytokines have been shown to be present in semen and the female genital tract (Figure 5.1, Wydooghe, 2017). It has been demonstrated that leukemia inhibitory factor (LIF) is present in the fallopian tube, and both embryos and tubal cells express LIF receptors. It is thought that LIF is involved in the implantation process. Addition of LIF to embryo culture media has been shown to enhance the quality of human embryos (Dunglison et al., 1996). Glycoprotein 130 (Gp130) is involved in mediating the effect of a range of cytokines and the addition of Gp130 to embryo culture media might have a positive effect embryo development in vitro (Hambiliki et al., 2013).

Animal studies have shown that the presence of granulocyte-macrophage colony-stimulating factor (GM-CSF) in culture media may exert a positive effect on embryo development, leading to significant interest in this molecule as a putative supplement to embryo culture. However, in a large prospective randomized study, the addition of GM-CSF to the embryo culture media revealed no overall positive effect on embryo development, implantation rates, or delivery rates. However, a post hoc subgroup analysis indicates a possible positive effect in the subgroup of patients with previous failed cycles (Ziebe et al., 2013). Indeed, in some of the early data on the mechanism of GM-CSF, it was concluded that one function was to suppress apoptosis in embryos (Sjöblom et al., 1999). However, whether suppression of apoptosis, which represents a mechanism by which an embryo may eliminate damaged cells, is of benefit is unclear.

A more recent prospective randomized study compared the outcome after culturing human embryos either in a standard medium or the same medium with addition of a mixture of cytokines (LIF, GM-CSF, heparin-binding epidermal growth factor (HB-EGF)). The addition of cytokines to the medium improved embryo quality (Fawzy et al., 2019), but as a mixture of cytokines were used in this study, it is not known whether the effect was due to an individual cytokine or the specific mixture used.

A few manufacturers add insulin to some of their culture media intended for IVF. The presence of insulin has been demonstrated to alter the profile of DNA methylation in mice embryos (Shao et al., 2007). DNA methylation is one way of regulating expression of genes and a change in DNA-methylation pattern is therefore usually accompanied with a change m-RNA profile and the proteins synthesized. Whether such effects present in human embryos remains unknown. Thus, the effectiveness of supplementation of culture media with growth factors and cytokines remains unclear.

5.3.3 Hormones

In vivo, the genital tract contains gonadal steroids, such as estradiol and progesterone. These steroids are key regulators of genital tract function and influence the molecules that are secreted into the fallopian tube lumen and to the uterine cavity. Addition of steroid hormones to embryo culture media has not proven to be beneficial. A major challenge of steroid supplementation is the difficulty of dissolving them in culture media, a feature shared with other lipophilic substances. In vivo, they are predominantly bound to carriers, such as serum albumin and sex hormone binding globulin (SHBG).

5.3.4 Vitamins, Trace Metals and Lipids

Some embryo culture media are very complex and reflective of products intended for continuous culture of mammalian cells. Such formulations can include up to 80 different components, including fatty acids, vitamins, iron chelators, trace metals, and intermediates in metabolism. It has not been shown that these

very complex culture media are superior to less complex media and it still unknown to what extent these varied components will affect development of human embryos in vitro.

5.3.5 Hyaluronic Acid

Hyaluronic acid may be involved in implantation and adding it to the medium used to transfer the embryo to the uterus has been shown to have a moderate positive effect on implantation rates (Bontekoe et al., 2015)

5.3.6 pH Regulators

In vivo, an important pH regulator is the $H^+ + HCO_3 \leftrightarrow H_2O + CO_2$ equilibrium. High CO_2 levels results in a low pH and low CO_2 levels in a high pH. Most embryo culture media contain bicarbonate and pH is regulated by the CO_2 concentration in the incubator. The CO_2 concentration should be adjusted to give a pH in the physiological range (7.2–7.4). One study on mouse embryos indicates a beneficial effect of having a higher pH at the zygote stage and lower pH from the cleavage stage (Hentemann, 2011). Addition of a pH indicator, such as phenol red, may offer a visual check on the pH of the culture media. However, phenol red is not an inert molecule and may change the metabolism of cultured mammalian cells (Morgan et al., 2019). It is therefore perhaps advisable to use phenol red–free culture media. In culture media that will be exposed to atmospheric CO_2 concentration, pH must be stabilized by buffers, such as HEPES or PIPES.

5.3.7 Non Physiological Additives

Follicular aspirates often contain traces of vaginal flora and it is reasonable to assume that most semen samples are not sterile (Kastrop et al., 2007; Koedooder et al., 2019). Antibiotics are, therefore, added to culture media, even though it has been demonstrated that presence of antibiotics may reduce embryo quality (Magli et al., 1996). These antibiotics are usually not manufactured with assisted reproduction in mind, and it can be a challenge for media manufacturers to source antibiotics that do not contain trace amounts of molecules, such as lipopolysaccharides (LPS), that will have negative effect on embryo development. It is a matter of discussion whether to add penicillin in combination with streptomycin or gentamicin or to use gentamicin alone. Semen and vaginal flora contain both Gram-positive and Gram-negative bacteria and since penicillin primarily works against Gram-positive bacteria, it is necessary to add streptomycin or gentamicin to also inhibit the growth of Gram-negative bacteria. Vaginal flora may include *Candida* species. Embryo culture media does not contain antimycotics, and if vaginal fluid is aspirated during oocyte recovery, the cultures may be heavily contaminated with *Candida* cells.

Some culture media contain EDTA which will bind divalent cations. In some animal models, the presence of EDTA will be beneficial for embryo development. For human embryo culture using modern culture media, it is not established whether the presence of EDTA is necessary for optimal embryo development.

Many embryo culture media contain surface tension and viscosity modulators to enable simpler handling of small volumes of media. The effect, if any, on the development of human embryos is unknown.

5.4 Oxygen Concentration and Antioxidants

In the fallopian tube, the oxygen concentration is around 5% and lower than in ambient air. In the early days of IVF, embryos were cultured with reduced oxygen concentration (Elder et al., 2015) while from the mid 1980s onwards many IVF-laboratories opted to culture embryos with ambient oxygen concentration. This change of practice was primarily for reasons of convenience and cost. Culture under reduced oxygen concentration often requires more sophisticated incubators, which are also more expensive to run. High oxygen levels may lead to chemical oxidation of a range of molecules important for cellular function. When culturing zygotes and embryos in 20% oxygen, it may be warranted to add antioxidant to the media. If this is necessary when culturing in reduced oxygen levels is unknown.

In somatic cells, oxygen concentration has profound effects on the gene expression profile, most likely mediated through hypoxia induced factors (Keith et al., 2007), and is also thought to play a role in the development of embryos (Kirkegaard et al., 2013). In human embryos, oxygen concentration is shown to influence the gene expression profile (Kleijkers et al., 2015). A relatively simple procedure changing from culture at below 5% oxygen, to 20%, and again down to 5% oxygen will lead to profound changes in the gene expression profile. It has been shown that the oxygen concentration has an effect on the embryo development rate and the implantation rate (Kirkegaard et al., 2013).

The long-term consequences of culturing embryos at an oxygen concentration four times higher than the physiological concentration is still unknown. It is now recommended to culture embryos under reduced oxygen concentration (Mantikou et al., 2012; Gardner et al., 2016).

5.5 Stability and Breakdown

Culture media slowly decompose after production. The amino acid glutamine is especially unstable and undergoes spontaneous deamination leading to accumulation of ammonium in the media. Ammonium is shown to have a negative effect on the development of bovine (Orsi and Leese, 2004) and human embryos (Virant-Klun et al., 2006). In most commercially available culture media, glutamine is bound to another amino acid in the form of a dipeptide and is thus more chemically stable. Protein supplements also contain glutamine and a comparison of commercially available culture media demonstrates that there is profound difference in ammonium accumulation during storage and incubation (Kleijkers et al., 2016b).

5.6 Single Embryo Culture vs. Group Culture

Coculture of embryos with mammalian cells was popular a few decades ago. Some groups presented data indicating that coculture with epithelial cells from the genital tract or human or animal cell lines was advantageous (Kattal et al., 2008). Use of human donor cell lines and of animal cell lines has been discouraged due to a potential risk of transmitting infectious agents. The alternative approach, establishing good cell cultures from the patient's own genital tract cells, was laborious and not always successful.

A potential alternative approach is to culture several zygotes and embryos in the same well or droplet. Embryos take up and metabolize molecules from the culture media as well as secrete molecules to the media. The hypothesis is that this paracrine effect is helpful for the group of embryos. A range of bioactive molecules, some of which are believed to be secreted by the embryos either as mRNA or proteins, as well as receptors for some of these molecules, have been associated with in vitro culture of human embryos (Figure 5.1). These findings suggest that human preimplantation embryos are involved in paracrine and perhaps even autocrine stimulation. Culturing embryos in groups rather than individually might increase development rates and embryo quality in culture of animal embryos (Wydooghe et al., 2014; Wydooghe et al., 2017). Concerning human embryos the data are, however, limited. Two relatively small studies from the mid 1990s suggests that group culture increased cleavage rate and embryo score (Moessner & Dodson, 1995) and pregnancy rate (Almagor et al., 1996). A more recent prospective randomized study also indicated a benefit of group culture of human embryos (Ebner et al., 2010).

A potential disadvantage of group culture is that it is difficult to trace the development of each and every embryo from the zygote stage until the blastocyst stage. Experience with time-lapse systems indicates that some embryos may form good quality blastocysts even when showing suboptimal cleavage patterns in the early stages. There is, however, a lack of good prospective studies comparing a strategy with group culture and embryo selection based only on blastocyst morphology, with individual culture where embryos can be selected both on history and morphology and/or morphokinetics. The relevant endpoints in such a study should be both delivery rate after transfer of the highest-ranking embryo and cumulative delivery rates after transfer of all embryos.

5.7 Summary

It is well known from animal studies that suboptimal culture conditions can have a lifelong effect on the phenotype of the offspring most likely mediated trough epigenetic changes (Fernández-Gonzalez et al., 2007). It has been demonstrated in several studies that the composition of the embryo culture media has an influence on the phenotype of embryos, the fetus and placenta, and the offspring (Kleijkers et al., 2015; Kleijkers et al., 2016a; Mantikou et al., 2016). However, we still have an incomplete understanding of the impact of embryo culture medium on long-term outcomes (see also Chapter 11), studies which will require extensive follow-up.

Studies to further understand the manner in which embryo physiology can be modified by the culture conditions are possible, although challenging. A major hurdle to such studies remains the lack of clear transparency of the composition of the different media products. Despite numerous reports outlining the components of commercial embryo culture medium (e.g., Morbeck et al 2017; Tarahomi et al., 2019), the manufacturers of culture media for human gametes and embryos do not make the exact composition accessible. It is, therefore, a significant challenge to link the effect on phenotype of embryos or children of a given culture media to its composition. This is unfortunate and scientific bodies such as the European Society for Human Reproduction and Embryology (ESHRE) have made a call for transparency concerning the composition of culture media for human IVF (Sunde et al., 2016).

References

Aguilar J, Reyley M. The uterine tubal fluid: secretion, composition and biological effects. *Anim Reprod.* 2005;2:91–105.

Almagor M, Bejar C, Kafka I, Yaffe H. Pregnancy rates after communal growth of preimplantation human embryos in vitro. *Fertil Steril.* 1996;66:394–397. https://doi.org/10.1016/S0015-0282(16)58507-0

Barnes FL, Crombie A, Gardner DK, et al. Blastocyst development and birth after in-vitro maturation of human primary oocytes, intracytoplasmic sperm injection and assisted hatching. *Hum Reprod.* 199;10:3243–3247. https://doi.org/10.1093/oxfordjournals.humrep.a135896

Biggers JD, Racowsky C. The development of fertilized human ova to the blastocyst stage in KSOM (AA) medium: is a two-step protocol necessary? *Reprod Biomed Online.* 2002;5:133–140. https://doi.org/10.1016/S1472-6483(10)61615-X

Bontekoe S, Johnson N, Blake D, Marjoribanks J. Adherence compounds in embryo transfer media for assisted reproductive technologies: summary of a Cochrane review. *Fertil Steril.* 2015;103:1416–1417. https://doi.org/10.1016/j.fertnstert.2015.03.010

Borland RM, Hazra S, Biggers JD, Lechene CP. The elemental composition of the environments of the gametes and preimplantation embryo during the initiation of pregnancy. *Biol Reprod.* 1977;16:147–157. https://doi.org/10.1095/biolreprod16.2.147

Brison DR, Houghton FD, Falconer D, et al. Identification of viable embryos in IVF by non-invasive measurement of amino acid turnover. *Hum Reprod.* 2004;19:2319–2324. https://doi.org/10.1093/humrep/deh409

Chatot CL, Ziomek CA, Bavister BD, Lewis JL, Torres I. Random-bred 1-cell mouse embryos in vitro. *J Reprod Fertil.* 1989;86:679–688.

Chronopoulou E, Harper JC. IVF culture media: past, present and future. *Hum Reprod Update.* 2015;21:39–55. https://doi.org/10.1093/humupd/dmu040

Dieamant F, Petersen CG, Mauri AL, et al. Single versus sequential culture medium: which is better at improving ongoing pregnancy rates? A systematic review and meta-analysis. *JBRA Assist Reprod.* 2017;21:240–246. https://doi:10.5935/1518-0557.20170045

Dunglison GF, Barlow DH, Sargent IL. Leukaemia inhibitory factor significantly enhances the blastocyst formation rates of human embryos cultured in serum-free medium. *Hum Reprod.* 1996;11:191–196. https://doi.org/10.1093/oxfordjournals.humrep.a019016

Dyrlund TF, Kirkegaard K, Poulsen ET, et al. Unconditioned commercial embryo culture media contain a large variety of non-declared proteins: a comprehensive proteomics analysis. *Hum Reprod.* 2014;29:2421–2430. https://doi.org/10.1093/humrep/deu220

Ebner T, Shebl O, Moser M, Mayer RB, Arzt W, Tews, G. Group culture of human zygotes is superior to individual culture in terms of blastulation, implantation and life birth. *Reprod Biomed Online.* 2010;21:762–768. https://doi.org/10.1016/j.rbmo.2010.06.038

Elder K, Johnson MH. The Oldham Notebooks: an analysis of the development of IVF 1969–1978. III. Variations in procedures. *Reprod Biomed Soc Online.* 2015;1:19–33. https://doi.org/10.1016/j.rbms.2015.04.004

Fawzy M, Emad M, Elsuity MA, et al. Cytokines hold promise for human embryo culture in vitro: results of a randomized clinical trial. *Fertil Steril.* 2019;112:849–857.e1. https://doi.org/10.1016/j.fertnstert.2019.07.012

Fernández-Gonzalez R, Ramirez MA, Bilbao A, De Fonseca FR, Gutiérrez-Adán A. Suboptimal in vitro culture conditions: an epigenetic origin of long-term health effects. *Mol Reprod Dev.* 2007;74:1149–1156. doi:10.1002/mrd.20746. PMID:17474101 DOI:10.1002/mrd.20746

Fredrickson J, Krisher R, Morbeck DE. The impact of the protein stabilizer octanoic acid on embryonic development and fetal growth in a murine model. *J Assist Reprod Genet.* 2015;32:1517–1524. https://doi.org/10.1007/s10815-015-0560-9

Gardner DK. Mammalian embryo culture in the absence of serum or somatic cell support. *Cell Biol Int.* 1994;18:1163–1179. https://doi.org/10.1006/cbir.1994.1043

The impact of physiological oxygen during culture, and vitrification for cryopreservation, on the outcome of extended culture in human IVF. *Reprod Biomed Online* 2016;32:137–141.

Gardner DK, Lane M. Fertilization and early embryology: alleviation of the "2-cell block" and development to the blastocyst of CF1 mouse embryos: role of amino acids, EDTA and physical parameters. *Hum Reprod.* 1996;11:2703–2712. https://doi.org/10.1093/oxfordjournals.humrep.a019195

Gardner DK, Lane M, Calderon I, Leeton J. Environment of the preimplantation human embryo in vivo: metabolite analysis of oviduct and uterine fluids and metabolism of cumulus cells. *Fertil Steril.* 1996;65:349–353. https://doi.org/10.1016/s0015-0282(16)58097-2

Culture and selection of viable blastocysts: a feasible proposition for human IVF? *Hum Reprod Update.* 1997;3:367–382. https://doi.org/10.1093/humupd/3.4.367

Culture of viable human blastocysts in defined sequential serum-free media. *Hum Reprod.* 1998;13 (Suppl 3), 148–159. https://doi:10.1093/humrep/13.suppl_3.148

Gardner DK, Lane MW, Lane M. EDTA stimulates cleavage stage bovine embryo development in culture but inhibits blastocyst development and differentiation. *Mol Reprod Dev.* 2000;57:256–261. https://doi.org/10.1002/1098-2795(200011)57:3<256::AID-MRD7>3.0.CO;2-P

Gardner DK, Phil D, Vella P, Lane M, Wagley L, Schlenker T. Culture and transfer of human blastocysts increases implantation rates and reduces the need for multiple embryo transfers. *Fertil Steril.* 1998;69:84–88.

Gómez E, Carrocera S, Martín D, et al. Efficient one-step direct transfer to recipients of thawed bovine embryos cultured in vitro and frozen in chemically defined medium. *Theriogenology.* 2020;146:39–47. https://doi.org/10.1016/J.THERIOGENOLOGY.2020.01.056

Hambiliki F, Hanrieder J, Bergquist J, Hreinsson J, Stavreus-Evers A, Wånggren, K. Glycoprotein 130 promotes human blastocyst development in vitro. *Fertil Steril.* 2013;99:592–599. https://doi.org/10.1016/j.fertnstert.2012.12.041

Hammond J. Recovery and culture of tubal mouse ova. *Nature.* 1949;163:28–29. https://doi.org/10.1038/163028b0

Hentemann M, Mousavi K, Bertheussen K. Differential pH in embryo culture. *Fertil Steril.* 2011;95:1291–1294. https://doi.org/10.1016/j.fertnstert.2010.10.018

Iritani A, Gomes WR, Vandemark NL. Secretion rates and chemical composition of oviduct and uterine fluids in ewes. *Biol Reprod.* 1969;1: 72–76. https://doi.org/10.1095/biolreprod1.1.72

Iritani A, Nishikawa Y, Gomes WR, VanDemark NL. Secretion rates and chemical composition of oviduct and uterine fluids in rabbits. *J Anim Sci.* 1971;33:829–835. https://doi.org/10.2527/jas1971.334829x

Iritani A, Sato E, Nishikawa Y. Secretion rates and chemical composition of oviduct and uterine fluids in sows. *J Anim Sci.* 1974;39:582–588. https://doi.org/10.2527/jas1974.393582x

Kastrop PMM, de Graaf-Miltenburg LAM, Gutknecht DR, Weima SM. Microbial contamination of embryo cultures in an ART laboratory: sources and management. *Hum Reprod.* 2007;22:2243–2248. https://doi.org/10.1093/humrep/dem165

Kattal N, Cohen J, Barmat LI. Role of coculture in human in vitro fertilization: a meta-analysis. *Fertil Steril.* 2008;90:1069–1076. https://doi .org/10.1016/j.fertnstert.2007.07.1349

Keith B, Simon MC. Hypoxia-inducible factors, stem cells, and cancer. *Cell.* 2007;129:465–472. https:// doi.org/10.1016/j.cell.2007.04.019

Kirkegaard K, Hindkjaer JJ, Ingerslev HJ. Effect of oxygen concentration on human embryo development evaluated by time-lapse monitoring. *Fertil Steril.* 2013;99:738–744.e4. https://doi.org/10.1016/j.fertnstert .2012.11.028

Kleijkers SHM, Eijssen LMT, Coonen E, et al. Differences in gene expression profiles between human preimplantation embryos cultured in two different IVF culture media. *Hum Reprod.* 2015;30:2303–2311. https://doi .org/10.1093/humrep/dev179

Kleijkers SHM, Mantikou E, Slappendel E, et al. Influence of embryo culture medium (G5 and HTF) on pregnancy and perinatal outcome after IVF: a multicenter RCT. *Hum Reprod.* 2016a;31:2219–2230. https://doi .org/10.1093/humrep/dew156

Kleijkers SHM, Van Montfoort APA, Bekers O, et al. Ammonium accumulation in commercially available embryo culture media and protein supplements during storage at 2–8°C and during incubation at 37°C. *Hum Reprod.* 2016b;31:1192–1199. https://doi .org/10.1093/humrep/dew059

Koedooder R, Mackens S, Budding A, et al. Identification and evaluation of the microbiome in the female and male reproductive tracts. *Hum Reprod Update.* 2019;25, 298–325. https://doi .org/10.1093/humupd/dmy048

Lewis WH, Gregory PW. Cinematographs of living developing rabbit-eggs 1. *Science.* 1929;69:226–229. https://doi.org/ 10.1126/science.69.1782.226-a

Lewis N, Sturmey RG. Embryo metabolism: what does it really mean? *Anim Reprod.* 2015;12, 521–528.

Lippes J, Enders RG, Pragay DA, Bartholomew WR. The collection

and analysis of human fallopian tubal fluid. *Contraception.* 1972;5:85–103. https://doi.org/10 .1016/0010-7824(72)90021-2

Lopata A, Patullo MJ, Chang A, James B. A method for collecting motile spermatozoa from human semen. *Fertil Steril.* 1976;27:677–684. doi: 10.1016/s0015-0282(16)41899-6

Macklon NS, Pieters MHEC, Hassan MA, Jeucken PHM, Eijkemans MJC, Fauser BCJM. A prospective randomized comparison of sequential versus monoculture systems for in-vitro human blastocyst development. *Hum Reprod.* 2002;17:2700–2705.

Magli MC, Gianaroli L, Fiorentino A, Ferraretti AP, Fortini D, Panzella S. Fertilization and early embryology: improved cleavage rate of human embryos cultured in antibiotic-free medium. *Hum Reprod.* 1996;11:1520–1524. https://doi.org/10.1093/ oxfordjournals.humrep.a019430

Mantikou E, Bontekoe S, van Wely M, Seshadri S, Repping S, Mastenbroek S. Low oxygen concentrations for embryo culture in assisted reproductive technologies. *Hum Reprod Update* 2012;19:209. doi: 10.1093/ humupd/dms055.

Mantikou E, Jonker MJ, Wong KM, et al. Factors affecting the gene expression of in vitro cultured human preimplantation embryos. *Hum Reprod.* 2016;31:298–311. https://doi .org/10.1093/humrep/dev306

McLaren A, Biggers JD. Successful development and birth of mice cultivated in vitro as early embryos. *Nature,* 1958;182:877–878. https://doi.org/ 10.1038/182877a0

Ménézo Y. Synthetic medium for gamete survival and maturation and for culture of fertilized eggs [in French]. *C R Acad Hebd Seances Acad Sci D.* 1976;282:1967–1970.

Ménézo Y, Lichtblau I, Elder K. New insights into human pre-implantation metabolism in vivo

and in vitro. *J Assist Reprod Genet.* 2013;30:293–303. https://doi.org/ 10.1007/s10815–013-9953-9

Ménézo Y, Testart J, Perrone, D. Serum is not necessary in human in vitro fertilization, early embryo culture, and transfer. *Fertil Steril.* 1984;42:750–755. https://doi.org/ 10.1016/S0015–0282(16)48202-6

Moessner J, Dodson WC. The quality of human embryo growth is improved when embryos are cultured in groups rather than separately. *Fertil Steril.* 1995; 64:1034–1035. https://doi.org/10 .1016/S0015–0282(16)57925-4

Morbeck DE, Baumann NA, Oglesbee D. Composition of single-step media used for human embryo culture. *Fertil Steril.* 2017;107:1055–1060.e1. https://doi.org/10.1016/j.fertnstert .2017.01.007

Morbeck DE, Krisher RL, Herrick JR, Baumann NA, Matern D, Moyer T. Composition of commercial media used for human embryo culture. *Fertil Steril.* 2014a;102:759–766.e9. https:// doi.org/10.1016/j.fertnstert.2014.05.043

Morbeck DE, Paczkowski M, Fredrickson JR, et al. Composition of protein supplements used for human embryo culture. *J Assist Reprod Genet.* 2014b;31:1703–1711. https://doi .org/10.1007/s10815–014-0349-2

Morgan A, Babu D, Reiz B, Whittal R, Suh LYK, Siraki, AG. Caution for the routine use of phenol red – It is more than just a pH indicator. *Chem Biol Interact.* 2019;310:108739. https://doi.org/ 10.1016/j.cbi.2019.108739

Orsi, NM, Leese, HJ. Ammonium exposure and pyruvate affect the amino acid metabolism of bovine blastocysts in vitro. *Reproduction.* 2004;127:131–140. https://doi.org/ 10.1530/rep.1.00031

Paternot G, Debrock S, D'Hooghe TM, Spiessens C. Early embryo development in a sequential versus single medium: a randomized study. *Reprod Biol Endocrinol.* 2010;8:83. https://doi .org/10.1186/1477-7827-8-83

Quinn P, Kerin JF, Warnes, GM. Improved pregnancy rate in human in vitro fertilization with the use of a medium based on the composition of human tubal fluid. *Fertil Steril.* 1985;44:493–498. https://doi.org/10.1016/S0015–0282(16)48918-1

Restall BJ. The fallopian tube of the sheep. I. Cannulation of the fallopian tube. *Aust J Biol Sci.* 1966;19:181–186. https://doi.org/10.1071/bi9660181

Restall BJ, Wales RG. The fallopian tube of the sheep. III. The chemical composition of the fluid from the fallopian tube. *Aust J Biol Sci.* 1966;19:687–698.

Rodriguez-Wallberg KA, Munding B, Ziebe S, Robertson SA. GM-CSF does not rescue poor-quality embryos: secondary analysis of a randomized controlled trial. *Arch Gyn Obstet.* 2020;301:1341–1346. https://doi.org/10.1007/s00404-020-05532-3

Shao WJ, Tao LY, Xie JY, Gao C, Hu JH, Zhao RQ. Exposure of preimplantation embryos to insulin alters expression of imprinted genes. *Comp Med.* 2007;57:482–486.

Sinclair KD, Young LE, Wilmut I, McEvoy TG. In-utero overgrowth in ruminants following embryo culture: lessons from mice and a warning to men. *Hum Reprod.* 2000;15(Suppl 5):68-86.

Sjöblom C, Wikland M, Robertson SA. Granulocyte-macrophage colony-stimulating factor promotes human blastocyst development in vitro. *Hum Reprod.* 1999;14:3069–3076. https://doi.org/10.1093/humrep/14.12.3069

Steptoe PC, Edwards RG. Birth after the reimplantation of a human embryo. *Lancet.* 1978;312:366. https://doi.org/10.1016/S0140-6736(78)92957-4

Summers MC, Bird S, Mirzai FM, Thornhill A, Biggers JD. Human preimplantation embryo development in vitro: a morphological assessment of sibling zygotes cultured in a single medium or in sequential media. *Hum Fertil.* 2013;16:278–285. https://doi.org/10.3109/14647273.2013.806823

Sunde A, Brison D, Dumoulin J, et al. Time to take human embryo culture seriously. *Hum Reprod.* 2016;31:2174–2780. https://doi.org/10.1093/humrep/dew157

Tarahomi M, Vaz FM, Straalen J, et al. The composition of human preimplantation embryo culture media and their stability during storage and culture. *Hum Reprod.* 2019;34:1450–1461. https://doi.org/10.1093/humrep/dez102

Tay JI, Rutherford AJ, Killick SR, Maguiness SD, Partridge RJ, Leese HJ. Human tubal fluid: production, nutrient composition and response to adrenergic agents. *Hum Reprod.* 1997;12:2451–2456. https://doi.org/10.1093/humrep/12.11.2451

Tervit HR, Whittingham DG, Rowson LE. Successful culture in vitro of sheep and cattle ova. *J Reprod Fertil.* 1972;30:493–497. https://doi.org/10.1530/jrf.0.0300493

Van Montfoort APA, Arts EGJM, Wijnandts L, et al. Reduced oxygen concentration during human IVF culture improves embryo utilization and cumulative pregnancy rates per cycle. *Hum Reprod Open.* 2020:hoz036. https://doi.org/10.1093/hropen/hoz036

Virant-Klun I, Tomaževič T, Vrtačnik-Bokal E, Vogler A, Krsnik M, Meden-Vrtovec H. Increased ammonium in culture medium reduces the development of human embryos to the blastocyst stage. *Fertil Steril.* 2006;85:526–528. https://doi.org/10.1016/j.fertnstert.2005.10.018

Wale PL, Gardner DK. The effects of chemical and physical factors on mammalian embryo culture and their importance for the practice of assisted human reproduction. *Hum Reprod Update.* 2016;22: 2–22. https://doi.org/10.1093/humupd/dmv034

Whitten WK. Culture of tubal mouse ova. *Nature.* 1956;177:96. https://doi.org/10.1038/177096a0

Whittingham DG. Fertilization of mouse eggs in vitro. *Nature,* 1968;220:592–593. https://doi.org/10.1038/220592a0

Wydooghe E, Vaele L, Piepers S, et al. Individual commitment to a group effect: strengths and weaknesses of Bovine embryo group culture. *Reproduction.* 2014;148:519–529. https://doi.org/10.1530/REP-14-0213

Wydooghe E, Vandaele L, Heras S, et al. Autocrine embryotropins revisited: how do embryos communicate with each other in vitro when cultured in groups? *Biol Rev.* 2017;92:505–520. https://doi.org/10.1111/brv.12241

Young LE, Sinclair KD, Wilmut I. Large offspring syndrome in cattle and sheep. *Rev Reprod.* 1998;3:155–163. doi: 10.1530/ror.0.0030155. PMID: 9829550

Youssef MMA, Mantikou E, van Wely M, et al. Culture media for human pre-implantation embryos in assisted reproductive technology cycles. *Cochrane Database Syst Rev.* 2015;20(11):CD007876.

Zhu J, Li M, Chen L, Liu P, Qiao J. The protein source in embryo culture media influences birthweight: a comparative study between G1 v5 and G1-PLUS v5. *Hum Reprod.* 2014;29:1387–1392. https://doi.org/10.1093/humrep/deu103

Ziebe S, Loft A, Povlsen BB, et al. A randomized clinical trial to evaluate the effect of granulocyte-macrophage colony-stimulating factor (GM-CSF) in embryo culture medium for in vitro fertilization. *Fertil Steril.* 2013;99:1600–1609.e2. https://doi.org/10.1016/j.fertnstert.2012.12.043

Optimal Handling Techniques for Culture of Human Embryos

Michael L. Reed and Thomas B. Pool

6.1 Introduction

The purpose of this chapter is to review some of the factors that influence laboratory and clinical outcomes, broadly under the heading of optimal handling techniques. Two principal environments are encountered – inside and outside the incubator. The chapter will address media buffers, gas atmosphere, timing and setting up culture or holding vessels, protection of medium performance, temperature relative to handling gametes and embryos, lighting, pH, incubation choices, and workflow. The importance of the interplay between these variables cannot be overlooked.

Defining optimal conditions and good handling practices requires dissection of processes and protocols. Many variables contribute to a solid laboratory foundation.[1,2] For accurate analyses, quality metrics must be established: New and existing laboratories should consult outside resources to develop or analyze performance goals. For example, a recent international workshop developed benchmarks for IVF[3]: Key Performance Indicators, Performance Indicators, and Reference Indicators were developed for oocyte quality, insemination practices, embryo culture, cryopreservation, and clinical outcomes. This report provides a disciplined starting point. (See also Chapter 10).

6.2 The Laboratory Environment – General Comments

6.2.1 Outside the Incubator

Outside the incubator, gametes and embryos are exposed to light, variable and nonphysiological temperatures and pH, airflow, and varying air quality. Exposure begins at oocyte retrieval and ends with embryo transfer and/or cryopreservation.

IVF requires varying degrees of micromanipulation, e.g., intracytoplasmic sperm injection (ICSI), hatching, and embryo biopsy. As technique complexity has increased, gametes and embryos are exposed more to the environment outside the incubator.

A single study mapped the time required by laboratory staff to attend to each of three IVF protocols: traditional IVF (350 min), contemporary IVF (520 min), and IVF that incorporates preimplantation genetic testing (780 min).[4] To place this study into context with this chapter, these estimated attention or personnel workload times highlight the additional time oocytes/embryos must be handled outside the incubator according to procedure complexity. Additional care is required to protect gametes/embryos during these extended work times.

6.2.2 Inside the Incubator

Incubators are classified as big- and small-box, benchtop small-chamber, and time-lapse (benchtop small-chamber incubator with a camera system) types. There are positive and negative features of each[5] (reviewed in Chapter 2). Oocytes/embryos spend the bulk of their laboratory existence in one of these devices, and some time out of incubation.[4]

6.3 pH, Buffer Choices, and Equilibration of Media

Managing stable levels of hydrogen ion and thereby a controlled pH in the embryonic microenvironment is essential for the efficient development of viable embryos. Dale et al. (1998)[6] demonstrated that extracellular pH (pHe) in culture media for human oocytes and embryos is a strong determinant of intracellular pH (pHi); the deleterious effects of pH oscillations upon cellular functions are well documented and summarized.[7,8] Of particular concern to embryologists are the adverse effects of pH fluctuations upon embryonic intermediary metabolism[9,10] and upon embryo growth, influences which are extended into and manifest in offspring.[11] That pH

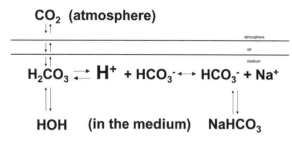

Figure 6.1 Stabilization of hydrogen ions with bicarbonate anions in culture media.

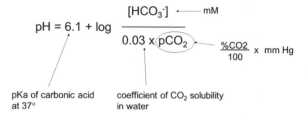

Figure 6.2 The Henderson–Hasselbalch equation. For color version of this figure.

has a direct role in meiotic spindle assembly in the oocyte[12] further elevates the possibility that oocyte aneuploidy is influenced within the embryology laboratory.[13,14] Achieving stable pH is simply a matter of understanding the buffer systems available to the embryologist, knowing how each system modulates hydrogen ion levels, and applying controls to each system appropriately.

6.3.1 Bicarbonate-Buffered Media

The generation of hydrogen ions and their stabilization with bicarbonate ions in culture media has been described in detail[15] and is summarized in Figure 6.1. Carbon dioxide is elevated in the culture environment, either in the incubator chamber or within a small enclosure, such as an isolette, funnel, bell jar–type lid, or microscope chamber. Carbon dioxide from the environment combines with water in the medium to produce carbonic acid, a weak acid that does not dissociate to completion. The products of this dissociation – hydrogen ions and bicarbonate ions – reassociate in the reverse direction to generate carbonic acid and these reactions rapidly reach an equilibrium, one that is defined by an acid dissociation constant, Ka. Sodium bicarbonate is included as a medium component, typically in the range of 20–25 mM, and acts to stabilize excessive ionization of carbonic acid. Stable hydrogen ion concentrations within the medium are then attained by adjusting the atmospheric CO_2 level that controls the amount of carbonic acid produced and, ultimately, hydrogen ion levels. Addition of more CO_2 into the atmosphere produces more carbonic acid, thus reducing pH, whereas lowering CO_2 levels has the reverse effect.

One principle the embryologist must keep in mind is that the amount of hydrogen ion generated depends upon the number of CO_2 molecules present in the atmosphere, and this number changes as a function of altitude. In other words, the number of CO_2 molecules present in an atmosphere of 5% CO_2 at sea level is not the same as it is at 1000 meters above sea level; therefore, the percent of CO_2 utilized is a relative term and adjustments must be made according to the altitude where the laboratory is situated. The easiest way to estimate the requirement is to use the Henderson–Hasselbalch equation – this is shown in Figure 6.2. Atmospheric pressure, expressed in mm of Hg, is used to calculate the partial pressure of CO_2.

A second important consideration concerns if and how the medium is supplemented with protein or any additional additives in the laboratory. Most albumin and other protein supplements are prepared and distributed in normal saline (0.9% sodium chloride). When an albumin solution is added, volume to volume, to produce a given working protein concentration, medium components are reduced in concentration by the same amount. This includes sodium bicarbonate and will reduce pH. For example, addition of 0.5 mL of a 100 mg/mL solution of human albumin to 9.5 mL of culture medium to yield a working solution of 5 mg/mL of albumin will yield a culture medium with a 5% reduction in all medium components, an effect that may be measurable in terms of buffer capacity. It is therefore crucial in quality control to measure the complete, supplemented culture medium for pH determinations in order to obtain an accurate reading.

6.3.2 Zwitterionic-Buffered Media

Working with bicarbonate-buffered media outside the incubator is labor-intensive as the surroundings must be controlled for appropriate CO_2 levels in order to provide stable and correct pH levels. A simpler alternative is to use media containing zwitterionic compounds, thus negating the need for additional CO_2 outside the incubator. Zwitterionic compounds are hybrid molecules containing both acidic and basic groups that can dissociate as either an acid or a base, depending upon the pH of the solution. In this manner, changes in pH are moderated, adding buffer capacity to the solution. One of the best known and most effective zwitterionic buffers employed in biological systems is N-2-hydroxy-ethyl-piperizine-N'-2-ethanesulfonic acid, abbreviated HEPES. This, along with 11 other zwitterionic compounds, was developed by Good et al. (1966) as an alternative to inappropriate buffers, such as phosphate buffer, that were inefficient and produced undesired reactivity or toxicity.[16] HEPES is a substituted taurine and provides excellent buffer capacity in concentrations of 20–25 mM. A second zwitterionic buffer, 3-(N-morpholine) propane sulfonic acid, abbreviated MOPS, has also been used quite effectively in handling media for oocytes and embryos, also in the range of 20–25 mM.

One important principle in selecting an appropriate zwitterionic buffer is to recall that the pKa of a buffer is temperature sensitive and that selecting a buffer where the pKa is closest to the desired working pH of the solution yields the maximum buffering capacity. The pH buffering range of HEPES is 6.8 to 8.2 with a pKa at 25°C of 7.48 and at 37°C of 7.31. MOPS has a buffering range of 6.5–7.9 with a pKa at 25°C of 7.2 and at 37°C of 7.02. When working at near room temperature, MOPS would offer better buffer capacity, but the choice shifts to HEPES at 37°C, given their respective pKas at those temperatures. One approach to negating the need to make individual buffer selections as a function of working temperature was developed by Swain and Pool (2009) who formulated handling media containing both MOPS and HEPES at concentrations of 10 mM each.[7] This concept of temperature independence through the formulation of a multi-protic buffer has been employed by several commercial vendors in both oocyte and gamete handling media along with vitrification solutions.

6.3.3 Equilibration of Media

Ensuring that bicarbonate-buffered media have been charged with a sufficient amount of CO_2 to produce the desired target pH for embryo handling and growth is a standard component of effective laboratory quality control. The time required for this process is dependent upon several factors including the culture volume and configuration (surface area), volume of oil overlay, oil type and permeability to CO_2, and atmospheric concentration of CO_2. Incubator chamber volume, gas recovery time, and frequency of chamber openings are also important in terms of knowing that the equilibrated levels remain constant. A recurring mistake made in many laboratories is failure to measure accurately or to use consistent oil volumes for culture. When this occurs, equilibration times may change for each dish prepared. Once the appropriate equilibration time has been validated for the culture system employed, a standard time of day can be set aside for this procedure, thus assuring repeatable buffer capacity.

6.4 Temperature

6.4.1 Outside the Incubator

Optimal handling and culture temperatures are still debated – benches, work tables, tube warmers, microscope surfaces, and inverted microscope stages are modified to maintain a desired temperature: Remember, however, that the temperature will not be static but rather cyclical around a set point. The cytoskeleton of oocytes is sensitive to cooling and wide and frequent fluctuations in temperature.[17] As routinely used, the target temperature for heated surfaces should be 37.0°C. Diligent monitoring is essential to identify hot spots, cold spots, and changes over time. Also, surface temperature may not be the same as inside a tube, or in a microdrop at the bottom of a dish. But the stability of the oocyte spindle apparatus with dissolution (chemical or temperature) and reformation is robust, and, with healthy oocytes, ICSI can be performed successfully at room temperature[18] Exposing oocytes and embryos to higher temperatures can be more damaging than cooling, e.g., compromising genetic expression.

6.4.2 Inside the Incubator

Incubation temperature for human oocytes and embryos has historically been targeted to 37.0°C, a presumed central measurement of human body temperature. In vivo temperature gradients across the ovary to the uterus have been documented in various mammals, suggesting that metabolic and other cellular requirements may vary according to site.[19]

Optimal incubation temperatures are species dependent, but there are only a few well-designed studies regarding incubation temperature and human IVF. Hong et al (2014) evaluated incubation at 36°C and 37°C.[20] Multiple incubators were used, and incubator stability was 36 ± 0.07°C and 37 ± 0.04°C. Fertilization and embryonic aneuploidy rates were not significantly different, but cleavage-stage cell numbers, blastocyst conversion, and "usable" blastocyst numbers were greater with incubation at 37°C compared to 36°C. There were no differences in per embryo implantation rates. Another study evaluated incubation temperatures of 36.5°C and 37°C and found no significant effects of temperature on outcomes, e.g., implantation rate or clinical pregnancy, in a large study population.[21] But while embryo cleavage rates were higher at 36.5°C, descriptive embryo quality was lower overall on day 3, and blastocyst conversion rate (formation and numbers available for cryopreservation) and descriptive blastocyst quality were significantly lower. Both studies concluded that despite the relatively narrow differences in culture temperatures, the target temperature of 37°C was overall the best choice for the human embryo.[20,21]

Incubators maintain a somewhat steady-state temperature, but the actual temperature, like gas phase transitions, will be cyclical. In addition, metabolic fluctuations could occur by extended or repeated periods of cooling (outside the incubator) and then rewarming (reintroduction to incubation). Dishes and tubes of various sizes and design, use of oil overlay, and movement to warm surfaces or tube holders can limit temperature fluctuations outside of incubation. Depending on incubator design, the time required for return to target temperature varies.[5]

Digital readouts on incubators can deviate from the "true" or actual temperature. While oocytes and embryos can tolerate (some) cooling, higher temperatures, e.g., over 38.0°C, inside or outside of the incubator, should be avoided. Choi et al. (2015) exposed one-cell mouse embryos to elevated temperatures (37, 39, 40, and 41°C) for short (8 hours) and long-term (96 hours) intervals.[22] Severe, short-term heat stress compromised early cleavage, and trophectoderm cell number and quality was diminished with long-term heat stress. Gene expression was altered, as were post-transfer fetal metrics. Youssef et al (2016) examined the culture temperature for mouse embryo culture.[23] Variable blastocyst development and hatching

blastocyst rates were observed at 36, 37, 37.5, 38, and 39°C. Blastocyst hatching was highest at 37.5°C, but combined development and hatching rate was higher at 37°C.

6.5 Osmolality

Osmotic stress and tolerance to stressors is development stage–specific.[24] Functionally, control of osmotic and pH stability begins at time of dish preparation.[25] Dishes with microdrops and oil overlay must be prepared carefully to prevent evaporation. It is recommended to turn off heated surfaces and air flow since both contribute to rapid evaporation, and the smaller the volume, the more rapid the evaporation. Upon preparation of multiple dishes, it is important to prepare one dish at a time, with small droplets being covered with oil immediately. This is a critical step: Immediate and downstream consequences can affect outcomes, particularly when using extended or uninterrupted culture methods.[26] The effect of incubation humidity on medium osmolality will be addressed in Section 6.7.2.

6.6 Light

6.6.1 Outside the Incubator

There is growing evidence that exposing oocytes and embryos to specific wavelengths of light, compounded by intensity and duration of exposure, can be detrimental.[27,28] Light sources include overhead and ancillary lights in the procedure room and in the laboratory as well as microscopes. If windows are present, plain glass may allow sunlight and heat to pass into the laboratory; tinted or appliance windows may be a better choice.

Specifically, near-UV/blue wavelengths (400–500 nm) should be avoided.[29] Dim the light sources when possible, although lighting must be bright enough to identify writing and colors, and to avoid obstacles about the laboratory. Fluorescent bulbs and microscopes may be fit with amber or green filters or acetate, but minimizing exposure is the goal – move dishes away from the light source whenever possible.

Preliminary evidence suggests intensity (lux) and duration of light exposure affects mouse embryo gene expression profiles, mitochondrial activity and cellular repair processes, maternal-to-zygote transition, and blastocyst conversion and morphology.[30] IVF-derived two-cell mouse embryos were exposed to control (no light) and experimental light (lux and duration of exposure) by a full-spectrum light source (visible light is 400–700 nm) fixed inside an incubator. After exposure (up to 6 hours) embryos were cultured in darkness. The authors conclude that intensity and duration of exposure "accelerated or accumulated the detrimental effects inside embryo cells." Note, however, that there were no details on culture conditions or temperature alteration inside the incubator due to the light source.

6.6.2 Inside the Incubator

Oocytes/embryos within incubators are not generally exposed to light. Time-lapse incubators are now common,[31] and light sources are designed to minimize duration of imaging while avoiding near-UV blue light (400–500 nm). Examples of imaging systems, with their light sources and exposure time, include the following: 1) EmbryoScope, 635 nm red LED, <0.032 seconds exposure; 2) PrimoVision 550 nm green LED, 0.005–0.1 seconds exposure; 3) EEVA 625 red LED, 0.6 seconds exposure; 4) Miri 635 nm red LED, 0.064 seconds exposure; and 5) Gena GERI green LED 591 nm, <0.05 seconds exposure. Even with multiple images taken each hour, total and controlled light exposure is measured in minutes.

6.7 Air

6.7.1 Outside the Incubator

The need for "good" quality air, meaning reduced particle counts, low to nonmeasurable volatile and other compounds, and a consistent mix of filtered recirculated and fresh air is not debated,[32] with the goal being limiting exposure of oocytes and embryos to compromised air.[33,34] Munch et al. (2015) observed decreased fertilization and embryo development for all embryos (ICSI and IVF), when, unknown to the laboratory staff, carbon filtration units were missing from the established air filtration system.[35] The negative effect of poor air quality was more pronounced for ICSI embryos than for IVF embryos. The negative effect occurred during the "peri-fertilization" period; oocytes and early embryos were more sensitive to suboptimal air quality. After installing new carbon filters, development returned to pre-impact quality metrics.

Optimal humidity within the working areas seems to be more personal preference than standardized, and there are no studies to suggest that laboratory or clinical outcomes are affected by room air humidity. Care must be taken to ensure dishes are covered, tubes are capped, and oil overlays are used when working with smaller volumes of media.

6.7.2 Inside the Incubator

The bulk gas component is nitrogen. Carbon dioxide is essential metabolically, and convenient for facilitating balance between bicarbonate and carbonic acid in culture media. Oxygen concentration is important from a physiological standpoint.[36] Quality of gases is also important – particulates, volatile organic compounds, and other "contaminants" must be kept at minimum.

Box-style incubators traditionally operate as humidity-saturated, where humidity levels can impact proper incubator function, maintenance of pH, and osmolality of media if dishes or tubes are used without oil overlay. Benchtop and very small chamber incubators may be humidified or dry.[5]

Lack of humidity, e.g., "dry" culture, has been the subject of several recent publications.[26,37,38] Elevation of osmolality of the medium occurs across the culture period despite dishes having an oil overlay. As the medium evaporates, it gains in osmotic potential, up to a 10% increase in some experiments, which will also change pH. Later-stage embryos do develop compensatory mechanisms,[24] but minimizing stress, e.g., by proper dish preparation, choosing a culture medium with a lower starting osmotic pressure, and changing or renewing the medium are all important considerations when culturing in a non-humidified environment.

6.8 Workflow

Laboratory design with engineering controls and choice of workspace layout has not always been an option for embryologists. Many IVF laboratories started as repurposed existing spaces (closets, office space, operating suites, etc.).

Regardless of design, the general flow and timing of events should be charted and controlled. A basic flowchart is useful to outline all of the steps encountered: In a simple IVF cycle, you have documentation, tube/dish preparation before retrieval, recovery/processing of oocytes, sperm preparation, insemination/microinjection, evaluation of fertilization, evaluation of growth, assisted hatching, embryo transfer, and cryopreservation of oocytes/embryos. Each step is an opportunity for appropriate or inappropriate handling, and correct or erroneous identification.

Witnessing, of at least critical procedures, is recommended, and there must be correct and thorough documentation of each step.

Each phase has specific requirements: personnel skills, timing of events, and environmental controls. Is there dedicated space(s) for each phase, or is there procedure crossover in the same shared space, which may cause mix-ups or collisions? As an exercise, the director, supervisor, and every technician in the laboratory should step back and observe each procedure from start to finish, breaking each phase down into components for critical evaluation. Process control is vital; each event or step, if not controlled, can have negative downstream consequences.[39,40] Workflow and laboratory design must be individualized.

6.9 Summary

The following list, while not exhaustive, may be useful when evaluating laboratory workflow:

- Proximity of equipment to individual workspaces
- Mobile vs. static workstations
- Incubators and workstations – low traffic, air flow directed at workstations or incubators
- Location of dedicated vs. shared workstations
- Minimal opportunities for extreme environment changes
- Minimal opportunities for accidents – clear foot paths, free of traffic and obstacles
- Minimal opportunities for misplacement of gametes, embryos – clear identification
- A team that works well together – communication is verbal and nonverbal. Avoiding conflicts in space and time. Awareness of personal space, workspace, and tasks
- Compartmentalization of techniques and technicians or "one person one cycle" workstyle; match skill level to procedures, and consider continuity of specimen identity
- Skilled floater person capable of filling in, or witnessing, or helping as needed
- Shift changes – notifications, hand-offs, sign-offs
- Communication – white board vs. daily worksheets vs. electronic calendar or all methods
- Staffing – 24/7, shifts, weekends, holidays
- Volume of procedures that must be accommodated; batching, random
- Disposables and consumables; having a good inventory mechanism, appropriate storage space (temperature and light), off-gassing, and adequate emergency supplies, including equilibrated media and oil in the event extra dishes are needed, or dishes become unusable.

References

1. Schoolcraft W, Meseguer M. Paving the way for a gold standard of care for infertility treatment: improving outcomes through standardization of laboratory procedures. *Reprod Biomed Online*. 2017;35:391–399.

2. Simopoulou M, Sfakianoudis K, Rapani A, et al. Considerations regarding embryo culture conditions: from media to epigenetics. *In Vivo*. 2018;32:451–460.

3. ESHRE Special Interest Group of Embryology and Alpha Scientists in Reproductive Medicine. The Vienna consensus: report of an expert meeting on the development of ART laboratory performance indicators. *Reprod Biomed Online*. 2017;35:494–510.

4. Alikani M, Go KJ, McCaffrey C, McCulloh DH. Comprehensive evaluation of contemporary assisted reproduction technology laboratory operations to determine staffing levels that promote patient safety and quality care. *Fertil Steril*. 2014;102:1350–1356.

5. Swain JE. Decisions for the IVF laboratory: comparative analysis of embryo culture incubators. *Reprod Biomed Online*. 2014;28:535–547.

6. Dale B, Menezo Y, Cohen J, DiMatteo L, Wilding M. Intracellular pH regulation in the human oocyte. *Hum Reprod*. 1998;13:964–970.

7. Swain JE, Pool TB. New pH-buffering system for media utilized for gamete and embryo manipulations for assisted reproduction. *Repro Biomed Online*. 2009;18:799–810.

8. Swain JE. Optimizing the culture environment in the IVF laboratory: impact of pH and buffer capacity on gamete and embryo quality. *Reprod Biomed Online*. 2010;21:6–16.

9. Edwards LJ, Williams DA, Gardner DK. Intracellular pH of the preimplantation mouse embryo: effects of extracellular pH and weak acids. *Mol Reprod Dev*. 1998;50:434–442.

10. Lane M, Lyons EA, Bavister BD. Cryopreservation reduces the ability of 2-cell hamster embryos to regulate intracellular pH. *Hum Reprod*. 2000;15:389–394.

11. Zander-Fox DL, Mitchell M, Thompson JG, Lane M. Alterations in mouse embryo intracellular pH by DMO during

culture impair implantation and fetal growth. *Reprod Biomed Online.* 2010;21:219–229.

12. Swearman H, Koustas G, Knight E, Liperis G, Grupen C, Sjoblom C. pH: the silent variable significantly impacting meiotic spindle assembly in mouse oocytes. *Reprod Biomed Online.* 2018;37:279–290.

13. Hassold T., Hunt P. To err (meiotically) is human: the genesis of human aneuploidy. *Nat Rev Genet.* 2001;2:280–291.

14. Swain JE. Controversies in ART: can the IVF laboratory influence preimplantation embryo aneuploidy? *Reprod Biomed Online.* 2019;39:599–607.

15. Pool TB. Optimizing pH in clinical embryology. *Clin Embryologist.* 2004;7:1–17.

16. Good NE, Winget GD, Winter W, Connolly T, Izawa S, Singh R. Hydrogen ion buffers for biological research. *Biochemistry.* 1966;5:467–477.

17. Wang WH, Meng L, Hackett RJ, Oldenbourg R, Keefe DL. Rigorous thermal control during intracytoplasmic sperm injection stabilizes the meiotic spindle and improves fertilization and pregnancy rates. *Fertil Steril.* 2002;77:1274–1277.

18. Atiee SH, Pool TB, Martin JE. A simple approach to intracytoplasmic sperm injection. *Fertil Steril.* 1995;63:652–655.

19. Ng KYB, Mingels R, Morgan H, Macklon N, Cheong Y. In vivo oxygen, temperature and pH dynamics in the female reproductive tract and their importance in human conception: a systematic review. *Hum Reprod Update.* 2018;24:15–34.

20. Hong KH, Lee H, Forman EJ, Upham K, Scott RT. Examining the temperature of embryo culture in in vitro fertilization: a randomized controlled trial comparing traditional core temperature (37°C) to a more physiologic, cooler temperature (36°C). *Fertil Steril.* 2014;102:767–773.

21. Fawzy M, Emad M, Gad MA, et al. Comparing 36.5°C with 37°C for human embryo culture: a prospective randomized controlled trial. *Reprod Biomed Online.* 2018;36:620–626.

22. Choi I, Dasari A, Kim N-H, Campbell KHS. Effects of prolonged exposure of mouse embryos to elevated temperatures on embryonic developmental competence. *Reprod Biomed Online.* 2015;31:171–179.

23. Youssef A, Kandil M, Makhlouf A, et al. Impact of incubation temperature on mouse embryo development. *Fertil Steril.* 2016;105 suppl:e45.

24. Baltz JM. Connections between preimplantation embryo physiology and culture. *J Assist Reprod Genet.* 2013;30:1001–1007.

25. Swain JE, Cabrera L, Xu X, Smith GD. Microdrop preparation factors influence culture-media osmolality, which can impair mouse embryo preimplantation development. *Reprod Biomed Online.* 2012:24:142–147.

26. Swain JE. Controversies in ART: considerations and risks for uninterrupted embryo culture. *Reprod Biomed Online.* 2019;29:19–26.

27. Ottosen LD, Hinkkjaer J, Ingerslev J. Light exposure of the ovum and preimplantation embryo during ART procedures. *J Assist Reprod Genet.* 2007;24:99–103.

28. Takenaka M, Horiuchi T, Yanagimachi R. Effects of light on development of mammalian zygotes. *Proc Natl Acad Sci USA.* 2007;104:14289–14293.

29. Pomeroy KO, Reed ML. The effect of light on embryos and embryo culture. In: Elder K, Van den Ven M, Woodward B, eds. *Trouble Shooting and Problem Solving in the IVF Laboratory.* Cambridge: Cambridge University Press; 2015:104–116.

30. Lv B, Liu C, Qi L, Wang L, Ji Y, Xue Z. Light-induced injury in mouse embryos revealed by single-cell RNA sequencing. *Biol Res.* 2019;52:48.

31. Armstrong S, Bhide P, Jordan V, Pacey A, Majoribanks J, Farquhar C. Time-lapse systems for embryo incubation and assessment in assisted reproduction. *Cochrane Database Syst Rev.* 2019;5: CD011320.

32. Guns J, Janssens R. Air quality management. In: Nagy ZP, Varghese AC, Agarwal A, eds. *In Vitro Fertilization: A Textbook of Current and Emerging Methods and Devices.* 2nd ed. Cham: Springer; 2019:29–38.

33. Mortimer D, Cohen J, Mortimer ST, et al. Cairo consensus on the IVF laboratory environment and air quality: report on an expert committee. *Reprod Biomed Online.* 2018;36:658–674.

34. Pontes BS, Resende MLP, de Castro EC. Air quality control on in vitro fertilization outcomes in assisted reproduction laboratories: a systematic review. *Hum Reprod Arch.* 2018;32: e000617.

35. Munch EM, Sparks AE, Duran HE, Van Voorhis BJ. Lack of carbon air filtration impacts early embryo development. *J Assist Reprod Genet.* 2015;32:1009–1017.

36. Gardner DK. The impact of physiological oxygen during culture, and vitrification for cryopreservation, on the outcome of extended culture in human IVF. *Reprod Biomed Online.* 2016;32:137–141.

37. Fawzy M, AbdelRahman MY, Zidan MH, et al. Humid vs dry incubator: a prospective, randomized, controlled trial. *Fertil Steril.* 2017;108:277–283.

38. Yumoto K, Iwata K, Sugishima M, et al. Unstable osmolality of microdrops cultured in non-humidified incubators. *J Assist Reprod Genet.* 2019;36:1571–1577.

39. Cohen J, Alikani M, Gilligan A, Schimmel T. Setting up and ART unit: planning, design, and construction. In: Nagy ZP, Varghese AC, Agarwal A, eds. *In Vitro Fertilization: A Textbook of Current and Emerging Methods and Devices.* 2nd edn. Cham: Springer;2019:9–20.

40. Morbeck DE, Duke M. Building the laboratory. In: Nagy ZP, Varghese AC, Agarwal A, eds. *In Vitro Fertilization: A Textbook of Current and Emerging Methods and Devices.* 2nd edn., Cham: Springer; 2019:21–28.

From Identification to Witnessing
Traceability to Ensure the Safety of the Embryo during Culture

Kelly Tilleman and Annelies Tolpe

7.1 Introduction

The most important purpose of embryo culture in the IVF lab is to make sure that the embryo can develop to its full potential in a safe and secure environment, and to prevent any errors that can lead to cancellation of the IVF cycle, or risk of other adverse outcomes. In a study by Sakkas et al. (2018),[1] including data from over 10 years and more than 35,000 fresh and frozen IVF cycles from more than 180,000 individual laboratory procedures, it was shown that the rate of moderate nonconformances was 0.23%. These failures are described as problems that negatively affect a cycle but not to the extent that the cycle is lost or severely compromised. Although the data from this study is reassuring and shows a very low rate of nonconformance during treatment, the most undesirable and catastrophic event that can occur in an IVF laboratory is a misidentification and mix-up of sperm, egg, or embryo. Embryo culture is a lengthy process that can last up to 6 or even 7 days in which the culture dish is manipulated regularly, sometimes on a daily basis, for purposes such as fertilization, embryo quality assessment, transfer, and cryopreservation. During these manipulations stringent procedures and protocols have to be in place in order to track and trace each and every embryo throughout the embryo culture. The ESHRE guideline for good practice in IVF laboratories includes a section on identification of patients and traceability of their reproductive cells.[2] Although traceability is part of the quality management systems in IVF laboratories today, there is not one system that is fail-safe.

7.2 Towards Effective Traceability

Traceability is key during embryo culture; however, when it does break down, it is important to have a system in place to be able to detect and find the root cause of the error or failure. Most of the time, many more factors than first identified are involved in a traceability failure. One problem-solving strategy that can be applied is the Ishikawa approach. This is illustrated in the fishbone diagram – a cause and effect diagram – created by Kaoru Ishikawa[3] (Figure 7.1); use of this makes clear how many factors can potentially be involved in a mix-up during embryo culture. The fishbone diagram can also be used for risk-analysis assessment, i.e., to identify the effects needed to obtain a desired result. Unlike trying to find the root cause to a problem or failure, the latter will show the identified factors that need to be controlled or in place in order to obtain the required outcome. As summarized in Figure 7.1, in order to obtain a traceability system during embryo culture, many factors need to be accounted for.

7.2.1 Method – Witnessing Procedure

Aside from a written protocol explaining the aim of traceability in your IVF laboratory, a specific method for identification and for tracing should be chosen. In most IVF laboratories, the 4-eye principle is still used. This manual double-witnessing procedure entails a double check by another staff member not performing the manipulation. A second person will double check the identification and labelling before the embryologist starts the manipulation or processing of the samples.[4] Aside from a double check before or during the procedure, a final check can also be performed at the end of a procedure. This final check is used to intercept adverse events that can be reversible upon detection, or that are not possible to detect until a procedure is complete.[5]

A traceability method entails more than verifying the identification label on the embryo culture dish to the patient protocol. Additional checking of the material through the microscope might be necessary in certain embryo culture process steps. The difference between the witnessing of the identification label on the dish (= dish check) and the witnessing of the embryo in the culture (= droplet check) should be

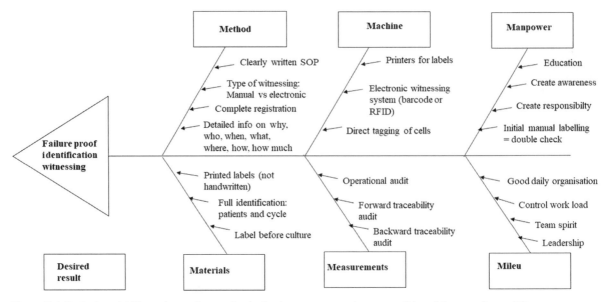

Figure 7.1 Desired result Ishikawa factors that need to be in place to come as close as possible to failure-proof traceability.

clearly described in the traceability protocol. When sequential media are used and certain embryos need to be transferred from the cleavage medium dish to the blastocyst culture dish, both a dish check and a droplet check is needed before the cleavage medium culture dish is removed. This droplet check verifies, for instance, that the right embryos are transferred to the blastocyst culture dish before any dish is discarded.

The double-checking approach does not only include the checking itself, but also the registration of the manual witnessing: staff members performing the first check and the double check must register this on a form or in the laboratory system. Preferably, the date and time should be recorded.[4,5]

A good traceability method describes:

Why to check: although it seems logical that double-checking is necessary in an IVF laboratory, still the rationale for the traceability needs to be described.

Who is checking: every staff member will check on their own that they have taken the correct culture dish in relation to the patient file they are working on. A double check will be performed by a second staff member (in the case of manual witnessing), before any manipulation to the embryo culture is done.

When to check: which process steps are vulnerable and pose a risk of misidentification and need double checking and witnessing.

What to check: For each check needed, a description of what to check is required:

dish check: the identification label on the dish in comparison to the file of the patient prior to any intervention

droplet check: verification of the embryo in the dish in cases of transferring embryos to other dishes

final check: this is a go/no go check: the next process step can be interrupted at this stage so that a mix-up is prevented. It is a double check that is executed at the end of a process step and before the next process step is started. It can include both dish check, patient file check, and/or droplet check.

Where to check: witnessing and control checks are registered in the patient file. A detailed description of the registration of the checks needs to be documented.

How to check: a description of the way checks are performed (manually or electronically).

How much to check: it is important to find a balance in the amount of witnessing checks that are performed. A group FMEA (failure mode and effect analysis) exercise to pinpoint the risks in the embryo culture will highlight the process steps where witnessing checks are necessary.[5–7]

7.2.2 Machine – Equipment for Witnessing

Aside from manual witnessing, electronic witnessing approaches and use of barcodes or radiofrequency identification (RFID) labels for identifying culture dishes have been implemented in IVF laboratories.[4]

Electronic witnessing systems have advantages over the manual double check performed by staff as they ensure that the embryologist works on only one patient's embryos at a time (and never more), and each process step is registered and controlled by the system. Furthermore, these systems monitor all the process steps constantly and a witnessing step can thereby never be overlooked; thus, embryologists cannot move on to the next step before a final check is performed.[8] Most of these systems provide a global traceability system that extends outside of the IVF laboratory and patients can receive a specific identity (ID) card that can be used during all clinical aspects of the fertility treatment. Because of these specific ID cards, patients will be aware of the traceability process in place. The study of Forte et al. (2016)[8] showed that patients felt comfortable with the electronic witnessing system and saw it as a tool to improve procedural safety in the laboratory. Interestingly, this study was performed at a time when a mix-up scandal in an Italian hospital was receiving a lot of media attention. Unique in its setting, this study showed that patients were aware of the possibility of mix-ups, and that information was given to the patients about how traceability and witnessing was performed. This created comfort and trust in the center where they were receiving treatment.

A more recent technology for tracing and tracking reproductive cells is direct tagging of the zona pellucida of oocytes and embryos by using silicone-based barcodes.[9] The purpose of this technology is to track and trace the oocyte/embryo during the in vitro embryo culture. The study shows that the development of the tagged embryos is similar to non-tagged embryos.[9] The engraving of an alphanumerical code in the zona pellucida by using femtosecond laser microsurgery is another emerging technology.[10] Although only tested in mouse embryos, the method does not seem to harm the development and viability of the embryos.

These experimental approaches still need extensive validation and although they are far from being introduced in clinical practice, it exemplifies the ongoing search for efficient traceability systems to avoid failures and mix-ups.

7.2.3 Manpower – People Involved in Witnessing

Staff require training and education to ensure that the traceability and witnessing protocol is successfully

executed. The very first step in all identification processes still involves a manual intervention. Therefore, initial labelling of dishes and other devices should always be performed under supervision, as this is the weakest link in the traceability process. Also with electronic witnessing systems, initial labelling through a manual intervention is required. Even if direct tagging of oocytes and embryos becomes a standard procedure, a double check during the initial step of the labelling of oocytes should still be mandatory.

Creating awareness of the importance of witnessing and formally recognizing the role of the staff in this crucial activity will generate willingness to support and adhere to stringent traceability procedures. It is therefore vital to engage the staff in risk assessment exercises.[6] Understanding the interaction of different factors, risks, and hazards that increase the vulnerability in the witnessing and how they impact the safety of the embryo and the patient is crucial.

7.2.4 Materials – Consumables Used For or Traced by Witnessing

Identification of embryo culture dishes must be performed by using printed labels. Handwritten dishes are prone to misspelling and misinterpretation.[5] A complete identification label with the full name of the patient(s), date of birth, and a unique identifier for the treatment cycle is recommended, as incomplete labelling can lead to misidentifications. Additionally, all dishes and relevant consumables must be labelled before being used. Record-keeping of all these consumables, tracking of batch numbers, and registration of expiry dates is mandatory for the traceability system and is necessary to complete the chain of traceability during embryo culture. This ensures the possibility of performing a comprehensive root cause analysis when a failure during embryo culture occurs. In addition, this information can and should be used to perform routine quality control checks and for analyses of performance indicators on the culture system and outcomes. It may help in explaining batch-to-batch variations and give answers to more subtle changes in embryo culture.

7.2.5 Measurements – Checking the Performance of Witnessing

The traceability procedure is also prone to failure, therefore it requires regular verification and the witnessing process needs to be audited on a regular basis. An operational internal audit will follow the complete witnessing procedure from the very beginning to the very end in the laboratory. A staff member, preferably someone working in the fertility center but not part of the laboratory staff, such as a nurse or a medical doctor, should meticulously follow the embryologists carrying out the witnessing steps according to the written traceability method (see 7.2.1 Method). An operational internal audit can show small differences in the execution of the witnessing in practice in comparison to the written procedure. The operational audit can thus reveal protocol drift but also disclose environmental and organizational aspects impacting the witnessing procedure.

Forward traceability audits start from a patients' cohort of gametes and traces them through the IVF process until embryo transfer and/or cryopreservation. Backward traceability audits start from the cryopreserved embryo and follow the traceability path back to the gametes. These audits are done in a documentary fashion where the registration and the completeness of the witnessing are checked.

7.2.6 Milieu – the Environment in which Witnessing Takes Place

Even when the factors above are tightly controlled and in place, the factor that has the most influence and poses the biggest risk on the traceability process is the laboratory environment. The IVF laboratory is a complex setting where different types of cells are processed in very different ways. Multistep procedures are performed by different operators and all have to work according to numerous protocols and procedures. Work load and limited time can lead to stress in the work environment[4] and impact on the efficacy of the traceability process. It is important for the staff to understand that only one task at a time should be performed and to take care of only one patient at a time. Full attention is required to perform procedures, including checks and witnessing steps, and distractions should be minimized or eliminated. A person dedicated to the witnessing steps can be helpful and will make sure that manual double witnessing is performed thoroughly even in situations of high workload. Although electronic witnessing can be a solution to minimize incomplete manual double witnessing due to distraction of a staff member, good day-by-day organization in the IVF laboratory is vital regardless of the witnessing system that is in place.

7.3 Summary

Mix-ups, involving patient mismatches and/or sample mismatches, do happen and are devastating to the couples involved.[11-14] A traceability and witnessing protocol is therefore a must in every IVF laboratory and is a crucial part of the total quality management system.[15,16] However, neither manual double witnessing nor electronic systems for traceability are fail-safe. Even in the future, if tagging of reproductive cells, or even biometric signatures on each individual embryo becomes possible, IVF laboratories will still be busy units with multiple samples being processed and manipulated by multiple staff members, all of which are risk factors. A good team spirit, shared responsibilities, and good leadership will help in creating a safe working environment where interventions and traceability witnessing procedures can be carried out with full attention.

References

1. Sakkas D, Barrett CB, Alper MM. Types and frequency of non-conformances in an IVF laboratory. *Hum Reprod.* 2018;**12**:2196–2204.

2. ESHRE guideline group on Good Practice in IVF labs, De los Santos MJ, Apter S. et al. Revised guidelines for good practice in IVF laboratories (2015). *Hum Reprod.* 2016;**4**:685–686

3. Ishikawa K. *Guide to Quality Control.* Tokyo: Asian Productivity Organization. 1976.

4. De Los Santos MJ, Amparo R. Protocols for tracking and witnessing samples and patients in ART. *Fertil Steril.* 2013;**6**:1499–1502.

5. Rienzi L, Bariani F, Dalla Zorza M, et al. Comprehensive protocol of traceability during IVF: the result of a multicentre failure mode and effect analysis. *Hum Reprod.* 2017;**8**:1612–1620.

6. Rienzi L, Bariani F, Dalla Zorza M, et al. Failure mode and effect analysis of witnessing protocols for ensuring traceability during IVF. *Reprod Biomed Online.* 2015;**31**:516–522.

7. Intra G, Alteri A, Corti L, et al. Application of failure mode and effect analysis in assisted reproduction technology laboratory. *Reprod Biomed Online.* 2016;**33**:132–139.

8. Forte M, Faustini F, Maggiulli R, et al. Electronic witness system in

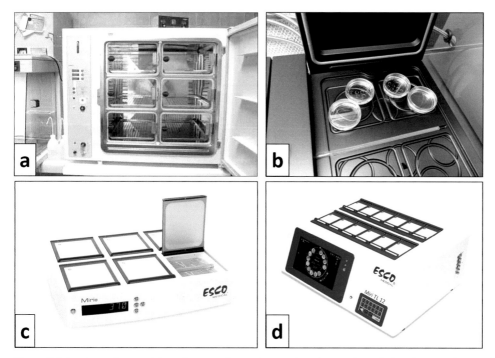

Figure 2.1 Incubators for overnight or longer embryo culture: **a.** large-box incubator; **b.** benchtop incubator; **c.** benchtop multi-room incubator; **d.** time-lapse incubator.

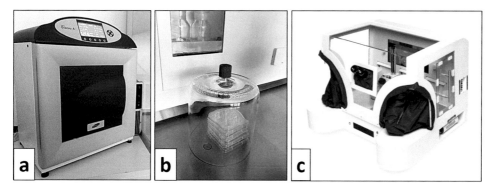

Figure 2.2 Holding incubators: **a.** smaller box incubator for sperm preparation; **b.** glass jar placed above an opening in the surface of the laminar flow through which CO_2 is introduced; **c.** closed workstation with controlled incubation atmosphere and integrated microscope.

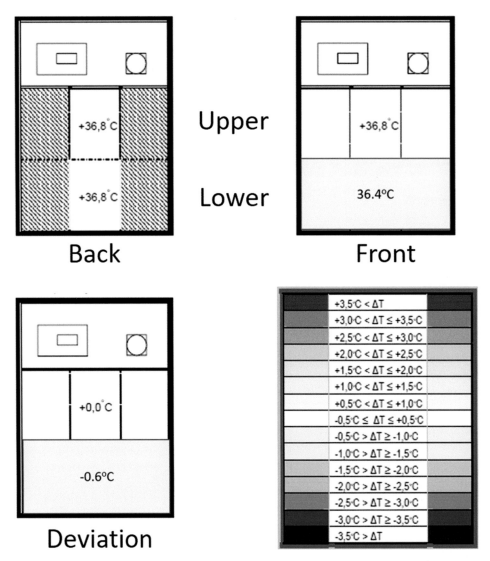

Figure 2.3 Incubator temperature validation report: **a.** measured temperature deep inside the chamber; **b.** measured temperature in the chamber near the door; **c.** deviation from the set temperature shown by the specific color of the deviation scale; **d.** color scale of temperature deviations from set point.

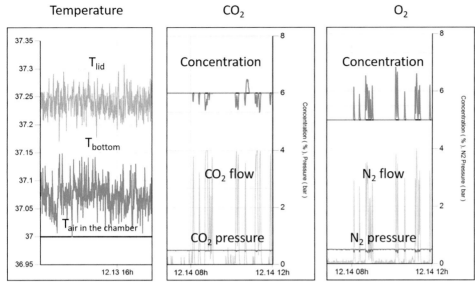

Figure 2.4 Display of continuous monitoring of physical parameters: **a.** temperature; **b.** CO_2, and **c.** O_2 concentrations.

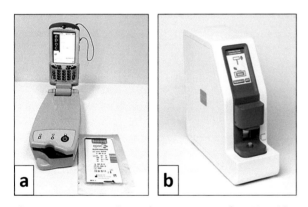

Figure 2.5 Measuring devices for measurement of: **a.** pH, and **b.** osmolality of incubated culture media.

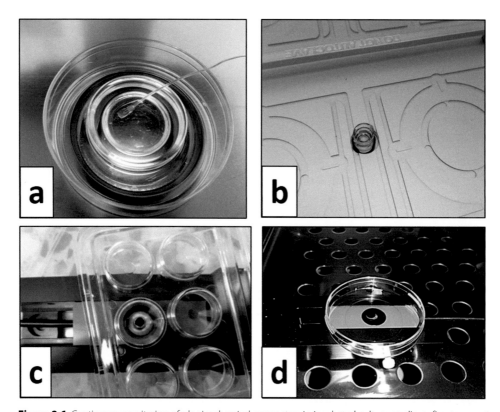

Figure 2.6 Continuous monitoring of physicochemical parameters in incubated culture media: **a.** fine temperature probe; **b.** integrated pH meter; **c.** and **d.** optical fluorescent measurement of dissolved O_2 in culture media.

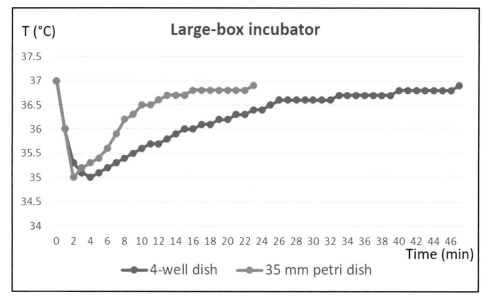

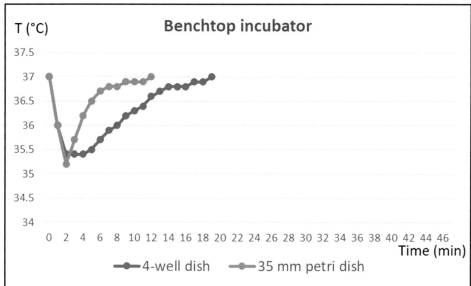

Figure 2.7 Recovery rate of the temperature of culture media after opening and closing of: **a.** large-box and **b.** benchtop incubators.

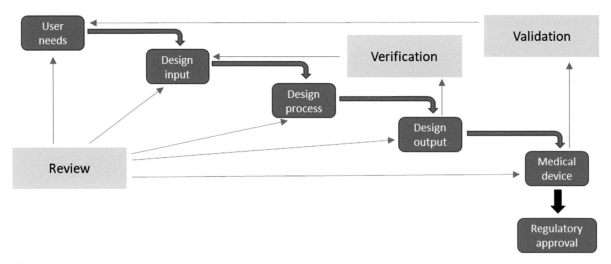

Figure 3.1 Process flow for medical design development.

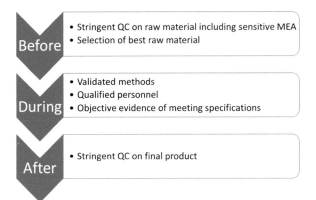

Before
- Stringent QC on raw material including sensitive MEA
- Selection of best raw material

During
- Validated methods
- Qualified personnel
- Objective evidence of meeting specifications

After
- Stringent QC on final product

Figure 3.2 Proposed flow for production of medical devices for ART, including raw material selection.

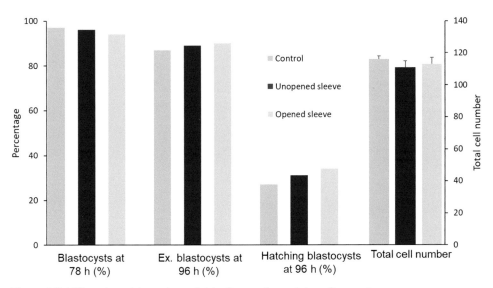

Figure 3.3 MEA results on labware immediately after opening or 7 days after opening.

Figure 3.4 ISO symbol for single use.

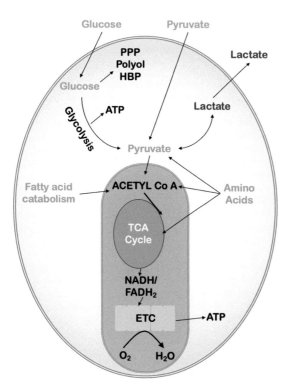

Figure 4.1 Simplified overview of energy metabolism. Glucose can enter the cell and take part in a variety of pathways; however, only glycolysis can generate ATP. The end product of glycolysis is pyruvate. This may be converted into lactate and excreted by the cell, or the pyruvate may be taken into the mitochondria and converted into acetyl Co A. Pyruvate itself may be taken up by the cell and used directly to make acetyl Co A. Acetyl Co A can also by synthesized by fatty acid catabolism or conversion of a number of amino acids. Acetyl Co A feeds into the TCA cycle which occurs in the mitochondrial matrix and produces the electronic carriers HADH and FADH2. These transport electrons to Complex 1 and Complex 2 respectively of the electron transport chain (ETC). The final reaction of the electron transport chain is the phosphorylation of ADP to make ATP and the reduction of molecular oxygen to water. This is the major cellular consumer of oxygen and is the reason that measurement of oxygen consumption is a good marker of mitochondrial activity.

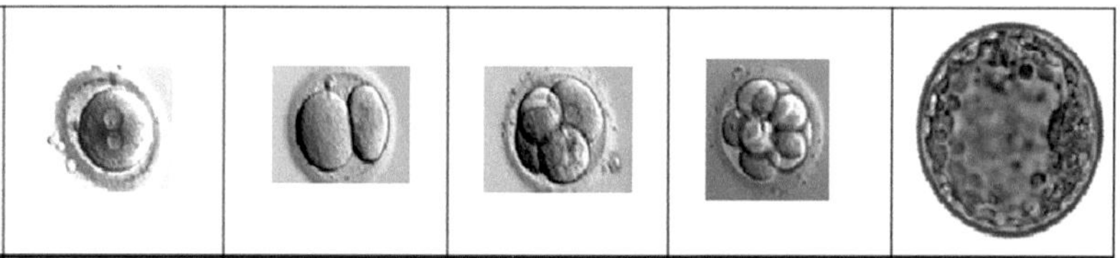

Glucose	Low/negligible consumption	Low/negligible consumption	Low/negligible consumption	Rising consumption	High consumption
Lactate	Modest production	Modest Production	Modest Production	Rising production	High Production
Pyruvate	High consumption	High consumption	High consumption	Falling consumption	Low consumption
EAA	Turned over	Turned over	Turned over	Turned over	Turned over
NEAA	Turned over	Turned over	Turned over	Turned over	Turned over
OCR	Low	Low	Low	Rising	High
Glycolysis	Low	Low	Low	Low	High
OXPHOS	Modest	Modest	Modest	Modest	High

Figure 4.2 Summary 'heatmap' of embryo metabolism. Increasing color intensity indicates increased activity, with red indicating substrate depletion and green indicating release. Blue represents 'activity'.

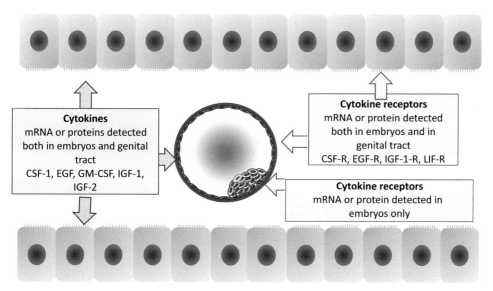

Figure 5.1 Cytokines and cytokine receptors detected in human genital tract and/or in human embryos. Adapted from data published by Wydooghe et al., 2017

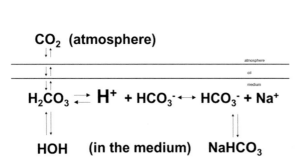

Figure 6.1 Stabilization of hydrogen ions with bicarbonate anions in culture media.

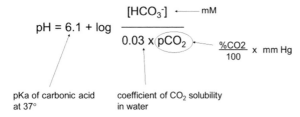

Figure 6.2 The Henderson–Hasselbalch equation.

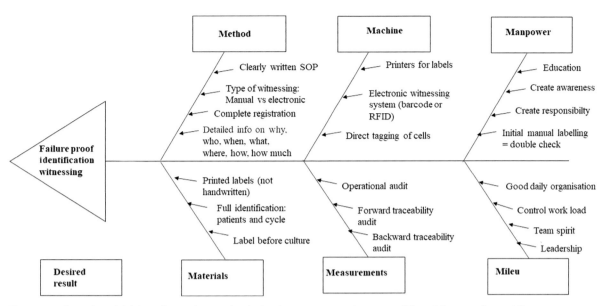

Figure 7.1 Desired result Ishikawa factors that need to be in place to come as close as possible to failure-proof traceability.

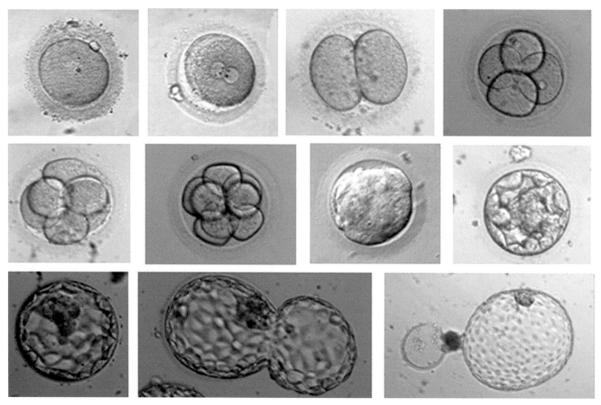

Figure 8.1 Preimplantation embryo development. (Photographs taken by the author).

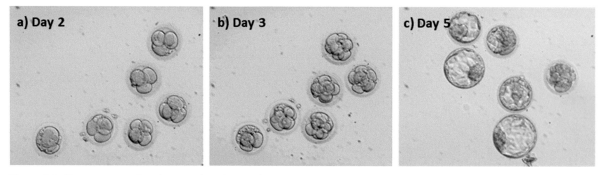

Figure 8.2 Pictures a patient's embryos as they develop from Day 2 (a), to Day 3 (b) to Day 5 (c). Embryo selection on Days 2 and 3 is hindered by the fact that all embryos look equally suitable for transfer. On Day 5, however, the formation of blastocysts allows a more accurate identification of the best embryos. (Photographs taken by the author)

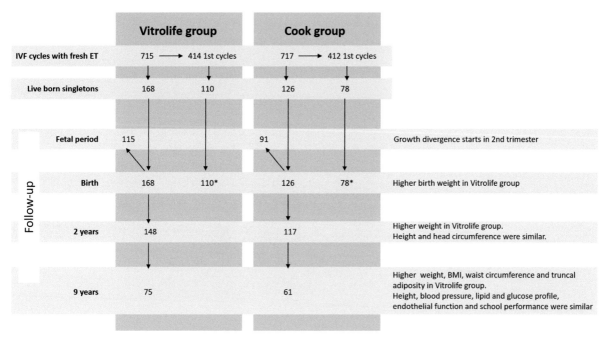

Figure 11.1 Flow chart and outcomes of a cohort of IVF cycles performed between July 2003 and December 2006, when the use of two types of culture media (Vitrolife and Cook) was strictly alternated between consecutive IVF cycles. Only a women's first live born singleton resulting from fresh embryo transfer was included for follow-up. The first paper for this cohort (Dumoulin et al., 2010) described birthweight differences in singletons born from women's first cycles (*). Later, the cohort was expanded with all singletons born. Retrospectively, fetal growth data from these singletons were collected. At 2 and 9 years, this cohort was approached for further follow-up. The numbers indicate the number of included subjects at each stage of follow-up.

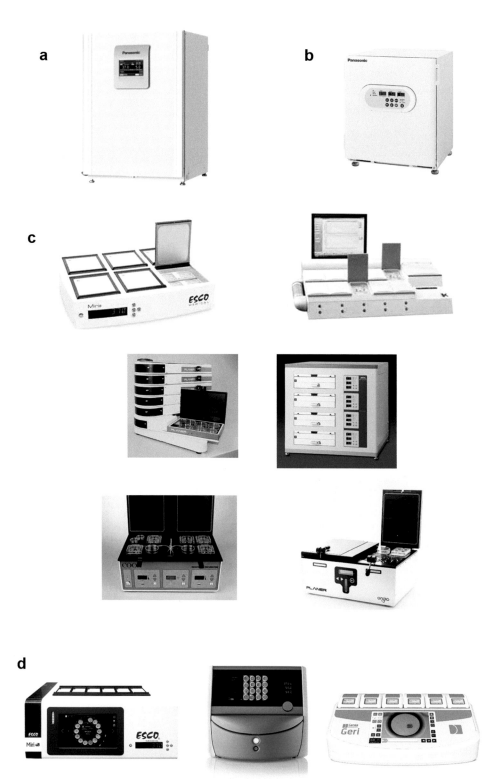

Figure 12.1 IVF culture incubators have evolved over time, reducing in size to units with individualized culture changes. **a.** Large box incubator, **b.** Small box incubator, **c.** various benchtop incubators, some with individualized chambers, **d.** time lapse incubators with individualized culture chambers. This evolution has results in improved growth conditions due, in part, to improved environmental stability.

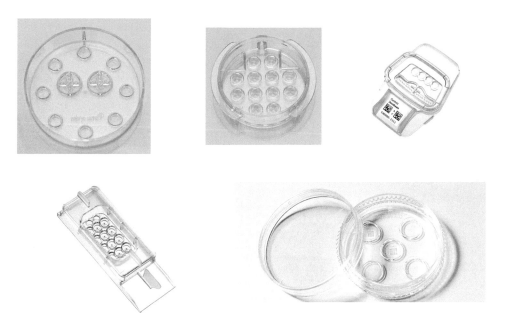

Figure 12.2 Various embryo specific culture dishes aimed at creating beneficial microenvironments and or permitting individual cell separation/identification. Embryos are increasingly being cultured in specific dishes tested for use with embryos for toxicity and customized to create confined microfunnels or wells rather than using generic cell culture/petri dishes and larger volumes of media.

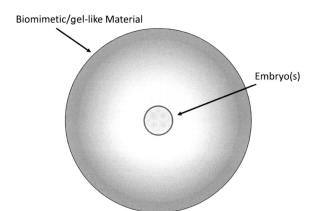

Figure 12.3 Three-dimensional culture approaches may offer a means of providing a more physiological approach to in vitro embryo culture by providing structural support and a more appropriate physical environment via different biomatrices. This method involves encapsulating cells into a bioscaffold or matrix material and has been used successfully for oocytes and follicles. Three-dimensional culture has not received widespread attention for use with embryos, but offers a means to provide structural support, a moist, rather than fluid environment, as well as present potentially beneficial molecules in an oriented fashion. However, 3-dimensional embryo culture does have unique considerations to address to facilitate embryo grading and recovery for subsequent uterine transfer or cryopreservation.

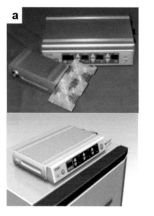
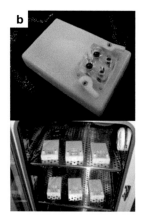
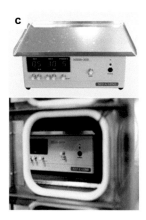

Figure 12.4 Representative images of dynamic embryo culture platforms that have been used clinically for human embryo culture. These platforms have historically required use of small or large box incubator and include **a.** tilting embryo culture, **b.** microfluidic culture and **c.** vibrational culture. Scaling down these approaches for use with smaller, modern benchtop incubators may provide an opportunity to improve upon current culture systems and facilitate more wide-spread implementation of this dynamic approach.

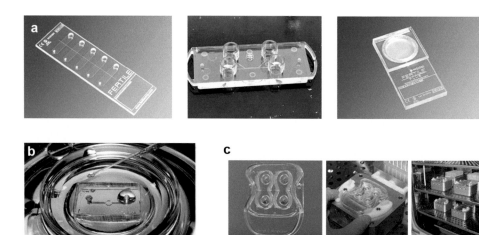

Figure 12.5 Various microfluidic platforms aimed at improving procedural steps involved in IVF have been examined, though most have not been widely implemented in clinical settings. **a.** Simple devices used for sperm sorting have received the most clinical use: semen is loaded into an inlet port and motile sperm collected from out an outlet port after traversing some arrangement of channels/obstacles to aid in sperm selection. While many experimental designs exist, at least two microfluidic systems have been tested on culturing human embryos: **b.** a simple static system and **c.** using actuated pins to drive fluid flow though microfluidic channels in a pulsatile fashion across embryos held in microfunnels.

IVF – patients perspective. *J Assist Reprod Genet*. 2016; **3**:1215–1222.

9. Novo S, Nogués C, Penon O, et al. Barcode tagging of human oocytes and embryos to prevent mix-ups in assisted reproduction technologies. *Hum Reprod*. 2014;**29**:18–28.

10. Ilina IV, Khramova YV, Filatov MA, Sitnikov DS. Application of femtosecond laser surgery in assisted reproductive technologies for preimplantation embryo tagging. *Biomed Opt Express*. 2019;**6**:2985–2995.

11. Dyer C. Human error and system failures caused IVF mix up. *BMJ*. 2004;**328**:1518.

12. Dyer C. Biological father declared the legal father in IVF mix up. *BMJ*. 2003;**326**: 518.

13. Rohde D. Black parents prevail in embryo mix-up. *NY Times Web*. 1999;**17**:3.

14. Spriggs M. IVF Mixup: white couple have black babies. *J Med Ethics*. 2001;**2**:65.

15. Mortimer ST, Mortimer D. *Quality and Risk Management in the IVF Laboratory*. 2nd edn. Cambridge: Cambridge University Press; 2015.

16. European Directorate for the Quality of Medicines & Healthcare (EDQM). Council of Europe. *The Guide to Quality and Safety of Tissues and Cells for Human Application*. 4th ed. www.edqm.eu.

Timing of Embryo Culture

Ioannis Sfontouris

8.1 Preimplantation Embryo Development

Following the fusion of the oocyte and spermatozoon and successful oocyte activation, preimplantation development begins with the formation of the zygote, displaying two pronuclei and two polar bodies if correctly fertilized (Figure 8.1). Embryo development continues with the onset of cleavage, i.e., consecutive mitotic divisions, leading to a major wave of embryonic genome activation between the 4- and 8-cell stages on Day 3 of development.

On Day 4, the embryo undergoes compaction, followed by cavitation and the formation of a fluid-filled cavity, marking the formation of an early blastocyst. The blastocyst continues to expand through mitotic divisions and the enlargement of the blastocoel, which occupies almost the entire embryo volume at the expanded stage by Day 5. The combined effect of increasing pressure from the expanding blastocyst on the zona pellucida and the action of embryo-secreted enzymes leads to a breach of the zona pellucida and the progressive escape of the embryo proper, until it hatches fully in preparation for implantation in the uterine endometrium.[1]

Development rate is considered the most important indicator of embryo viability.[2] For example, on Day 3 (68 ± 1 hour post insemination), embryos with ≤6 cells are considered slow, embryos with 7–9 cells normal, and embryos with ≥10 cells are considered accelerated.[3] There is evidence to suggest that too slow or too fast embryo cleavage has a negative impact on implantation rate. In addition, embryos with deviations in cleavage rate are associated with a higher incidence of chromosomal abnormalities compared with normally developing embryos.[4]

Standardized timing of evaluations performed at set time points (hours post insemination/microinjection) enables development rates and results to be compared between different embryo cohorts and different laboratories.[3] (See Table 8.1). However, it must be noted that these recommendations were made based on static observations of embryos once or twice daily. The introduction of time-lapse technology has provided a wealth of new information. A better knowledge of timings and intervals between cell divisions, as well as the possibility of identifying abnormal cleavage patterns, such as direct or reverse cleavage, are likely to lead to a revision of the criteria for embryo assessment.

8.2 Embryo Culture and Timing of Transfer

The study of mammalian preimplantation embryos in vitro became possible as early as the mid-1950s. The first culture medium specifically devised for mammalian (mouse) embryos was described by Whitten in 1956.[5] Subsequently, the pioneering work of McLaren and Biggers in 1958 reported that 8-cell mouse embryos cultured until the blastocyst stage would develop into normal young after transfer to the uterus of surrogate mothers.[6] Despite those early advances in mouse embryo culture, extended culture of human embryos remained challenging for several years. Initial attempts of culturing human embryos to the blastocyst stage in simplified media resulted in acceptable blastocyst formation rates, but in disappointingly low implantation and pregnancy rates. For this reason, transfer of embryos on day 2 or day 3 remained standard practice in human IVF for almost two decades.[8]

The first reliable approach for successful extended culture of human embryos depended on the use of sequential culture media, which were designed to meet the changing metabolic and nutritional requirements of the developing embryo. However, there is now renewed interest in the use of a single medium to

Table 8.1 Recommendations of the Istanbul Consensus regarding the timing of observation of fertilized oocytes and embryos, and the expected stage of development at each time point.[3]

Type of observation	Timing (h post insemination)	Expected stage of development
Fertilization check	17 ± 1	Pronuclear (PN) stage
Syngamy check	23 ± 1	Expect 50% to be in syngamy (up to 20% may be at the 2-cell stage)
Early cleavage check	26 ± 1 post ICSI 28 ± 1 post IVF	2-cell stage
Day 2 embryo assessment	44 ± 1	4-cell stage
Day 3 embryo assessment	68 ± 1	8-cell stage
Day 4 embryo assessment	92 ± 2	Morula
Day 5 embryo assessment	116 ± 2	Blastocyst

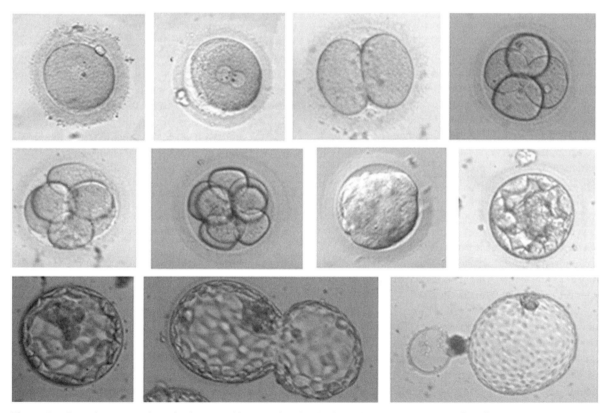

Figure 8.1 Preimplantation embryo development. (Photographs taken by the author). For color version of this figure. Please refer color plate section.

support development of the embryo during the entire preimplantation period, based on a single formulation. Especially with the implementation of closed culture with time-lapse imaging, single culture media is again gaining ground. Both single and sequential media have been shown to be equally efficient in supporting embryo development to the blastocyst stage, and both approaches seem to be associated with similar reproductive outcomes.[10] (See discussion in Chapter 5).

Certainly, blastocyst culture is more technically demanding compared to Day 2/3 culture, and there are several laboratory aspects that should be considered apart from the culture medium. Extended culture up to the blastocyst stage requires greater incubator capacity, which will depend on the number of cycles each clinic accommodates. Moreover, moving embryos to fresh medium on day 3, if sequential media are used, can increase workload in busy laboratories. In addition, air filtration, pH monitoring of culture media, and use of low oxygen are of crucial importance for a successful blastocyst transfer program.

The ability to grow human embryos until the blastocyst stage using new generation media has provided clinics with more flexibility, as now embryo transfers can be performed on all days of preimplantation development. Embryos are usually transferred either at the cleavage stage (on Day 2 or 3) or at the blastocyst stage (on Day 5). Current evidence suggests that blastocyst transfer of Day 6 is associated with lower clinical pregnancy and live birth rates than Day 5, especially for fresh transfers.[11] Therefore, it is suggested that slow developing embryos that form a blastocyst on Day 6 are cryopreserved, and transferred in a subsequent frozen replacement cycle on Day 5.[12] At present, morula transfer on Day 4 is less common (see discussion in 8.3 The Morula Stage.)

Blastocyst transfer is becoming more popular mainly because it offers several advantages, discussed below, and is theoretically associated with an increased probability of implantation compared to cleavage stage transfer. However, there is still a debate regarding the comparative efficacy of cleavage and blastocyst culture per oocyte pick-up, and in addition some concerns have been expressed regarding the effect of extended culture on perinatal outcomes.

8.2.1 Cleavage-Stage and Blastocyst Transfer

8.2.1.1 Embryo Selection

The cohort of oocytes retrieved from a patient following controlled ovarian stimulation is quite heterogeneous in terms of maturity and developmental competence. Consequently, the resulting embryos have a marked variability in their developmental and implantation potential. Therefore, there is a constant challenge for embryologists to accurately distinguish good quality embryos and select those for transfer. In this respect, embryo morphology assessment has historically been the first line tool for embryo selection. However, morphological assessment is subjective and is characterized by high intra- and inter-operator variability.[13] Moreover, embryo morphology on Days 2–3 has been shown to have limited ability to predict blastocyst formation on Day 5 (Figure 8.2).[14]

Blastocyst formation rates usually range from 40% to 60%, meaning that not all embryos have the potential to form a blastocyst.[10] Therefore, extending culture to Day 5 is considered to represent a mechanism for self-selection of embryos with higher developmental competence. The blastocyst stage reflects embryos that have successfully made the transition from maternal dependence to embryonic genome activation, while there is also evidence that blastocysts are associated with a reduced incidence of aneuploidies compared to cleavage-stage embryos.[15]

8.2.1.2 Single Embryo Transfer and Reduction of Multiple Pregnancies

Faced with our current inability to accurately identify the single best embryo for transfer from a patient's cohort, in some cases two or more embryos are transferred. As a result, the risk of multiple pregnancies is increased. Multiple pregnancy is the most serious complication of IVF as it carries a higher chance of miscarriage, perinatal mortality, cerebral palsy, hypertension, preeclampsia, gestational diabetes and the need for a caesarean birth.

Moreover, in the UK, it is reported that the average cost to the NHS is £13,959 for a twin birth, compared to £4,892 for a singleton birth. The percentage of multiple pregnancies from IVF in the UK has seen a progressive decline because of changes in policy and the implementation of elective single

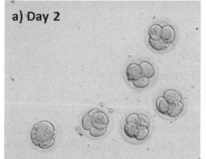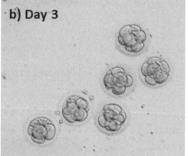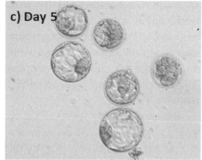

Figure 8.2 Pictures a patient's embryos as they develop from Day 2 (a), to Day 3 (b) to Day 5 (c). Embryo selection on Days 2 and 3 is hindered by the fact that all embryos look equally suitable for transfer. On Day 5, however, the formation of blastocysts allows a more accurate identification of the best embryos. (Photographs taken by the author).

embryo transfer (eSET). This decrease clearly needs to be sustained. A recent report issued from the Human Fertilization and Embryology Authority (HFEA) shows that for every 10% reduction in the current rate of multiple births, £15 million could be saved by the NHS.

The ultimate goal of efficient and accurate embryo selection is therefore to maximize the probability of selecting the embryo with highest potential first. To this end, improved embryo selection, facilitated by blastocyst culture, may promote the use of eSET, by making feasible the transfer of a single embryo without reducing the patients' chances of a successful pregnancy.

Current evidence suggests that in good-prognosis patients, transfer of a single blastocyst significantly decreases the incidence of multiple pregnancy, while maintaining pregnancy rates comparable to those following double blastocyst transfer.[16] In addition, the decline in multiple birth rates has been shown to have a positive impact on the health of the offspring. Follow-up studies show that perinatal risks for ART children has decreased and overall health has improved.[17]

8.2.1.3 Embryo–Uterine Synchronization

The efficiency and flexibility of human IVF has benefited greatly from the ability to transfer embryos at all preimplantation stages (cleavage-stage or blastocyst) to the uterus. It should be noted that, in vivo, cleavage stage embryos reside in the fallopian tube and not in the uterus. Interestingly, in domestic and other mammalian species, transfer of cleavage stage embryos into the uterus results in impaired development and

low pregnancy rates, thus necessitating transfer at the morula or blastocyst stage.

In humans, however, transfer of cleavage stage embryos to the uterus does not appear to compromise their development or their ability to implant. Nevertheless, there remains a theoretical advantage that transfer of a blastocyst may allow for a more physiological synchronization of the embryo stage and the uterine environment, possibly leading to improved implantation rates.[8]

8.2.1.4 Embryo Biopsy for Preimplantation Genetic Testing

Currently, all preimplantation genetic testing (PGT) programs involve performing an embryo biopsy. Biopsy can be performed by removal of one or two polar bodies, respectively, from the unfertilized oocyte or the zygote, blastomere removal from Day 3 embryos, or removal of five to ten trophectoderm cells at the blastocyst stage during Days 5–7 post-insemination.[18]

Cleavage stage biopsy involves the removal of a single blastomere of a Day 3 embryo that has at least six blastomeres up to precompaction stages. At these stages, blastomeres have the potential to contribute to the embryo proper since they have not yet committed to either the inner cell mass or trophectoderm. It is possible to detect meiotic errors, but mitotic errors leading to chromosomal mosaicism cannot be identified, and the amount of DNA obtained from a single cell is limited.

Following biopsy, embryos are either further cultured to the blastocyst stage while waiting for the genetic result or are cryopreserved. This latter approach is characterized by increased laboratory workload, as a high number of Day 3 embryos are biopsied, whose potential to develop to the blastocyst stage is still unknown. A negative impact of cleavage stage biopsy on embryo developmental competence has been suggested,[19] especially if two cells are removed.[20]

Blastocyst biopsy involves the removal of 5 to 10 trophectoderm cells. These cells are destined to give rise to the placenta and the extraembryonic membranes and not the embryo proper, thus theoretically inflicting lower impact on the fetus, which originates from the inner cell mass.

While cleavage-stage biopsy was originally the most widely practiced form of embryo biopsy,[18] its clinical use has now been reduced. Modern PGT strategies involve biopsy at the blastocyst stage followed by comprehensive chromosome screening and possibly combined with vitrification.[19] Blastocyst biopsy is the most widely adopted technique, as it provides higher reliability by the analysis of a higher number of cells, ability to detect chromosome mosaicisms, is associated with lower laboratory workload by biopsying fewer embryos, and is less sensitive to possible embryo damage compared to cleavage-stage biopsy.

8.2.1.5 Embryo Cryopreservation

Embryo cryopreservation has become a vital key component of IVF programs, allowing several embryo transfers from the same oocyte retrieval cycle, leading to an increase in cumulative pregnancy rates. Extended culture to the blastocyst stage and blastocyst cryopreservation has a central role in modern ART strategies. Although slow-freezing seemed to compromise blastocyst cryosurvival, as indicated by lower cumulative pregnancy rates,[22] blastocyst vitrification offers excellent survival rates.[23] Interestingly, there is only one available randomized control trial (RCT) comparing cleavage-stage and blastocyst cryopreservation using vitrification.[24] This study reported significantly higher cumulative pregnancy rates in the blastocyst stage group (Day 3 freezing: 43.3% vs. Day 5 freezing: 56.8%).

The success rates of blastocyst vitrification have significantly increased the efficiency of IVF and have transformed modern clinical practice.[25] Furthermore, successful cryopreservation is essential for an effective eSET program, segmentation of treatment to prevent ovarian hyperstimulation syndrome by employing a freeze-all policy,[26] and implementation of modern PGT strategies.[21]

2.1.6 Monitoring of Ovarian Hyperstimulation Syndrome

Ovarian hyperstimulation syndrome (OHSS) is a serious and potentially life-threatening iatrogenic complication of ovarian stimulation. OHSS is triggered by human chorionic gonadotrophin (hCG), which induces excessive ovarian secretion of angiogenic factors, resulting in increased vascular permeability, fluid shift to the third space, and ascites accumulation in the third space and peritoneum. Early-onset OHSS occurs within 5 days after oocyte retrieval and is classified in mild, moderate, and severe forms.[27]

Generally, in high-risk for OHSS patients, culture to the blastocyst stage is recommended and allows better clinical evaluation of the patient, with the possibility of embryo transfer cancellation, in case severe OHSS develops by Day 5. Usually, patients at high risk for OHSS are women with a good ovarian reserve, who yield high numbers of oocytes and embryos and are therefore suitable for blastocyst culture. Blastocyst transfer may be performed if severe OHSS is not diagnosed on Day 5. However, these patients should be informed about the probability of late pregnancy-induced OHSS and ideally be offered a freeze-all option.[28]

8.2.2 Outcomes after Cleavage-Stage and Blastocyst Transfer

In any IVF intervention, the day of transfer should be selected to maximize the chance of pregnancy and live birth per transfer and also per oocyte retrieval (cumulative live birth). However, the overall efficiency of which day of transfer to select is not unambiguously clear.

The most recent Cochrane review,[22] which included 27 RCTs of women undergoing autologous IVF/ICSI cycles, reported low-quality evidence for higher live-birth rate after blastocyst transfer (odds ratio (OR) 1.48, 95% confidence interval (CI) 1.20–1.82; 13 RCTs, 1,630 women). However, this beneficial effect on live-birth rate was not maintained when restricted to studies with a low risk of bias. There was moderate evidence for higher clinical pregnancy rate after blastocyst transfers (OR 1.30, 95% CI 1.14–1.47; 27 RCTs, 4031 women), and the effect was still present when restricted to studies with a low risk of bias.

Cumulative pregnancy rate was similar between cleavage-stage and blastocyst transfer (OR 0.89, 95% CI 0.64–1.22; 5 RCTs, 632 women) although the quality of evidence was graded as very low. Similarly, there were there were no differences in multiple pregnancy or miscarriage between the two groups.

According to the American Society for Reproductive Medicine recommendation, although there is evidence suggesting that blastocyst transfer may yield better rates of clinical pregnancy and live birth, more studies are needed to incorporate outcomes for single-embryo transfer, cumulative pregnancy rate, and PGT.[16]

A subsequent meta-analysis with different methodology and study inclusion criteria identified 12 eligible RCTs, involving a total 1200 women undergoing blastocyst transfer and 1218 undergoing cleavage-stage transfer.[29] The meta-analysis showed no significant differences in ongoing/live birth, clinical pregnancy, miscarriage, or cumulative pregnancy rates between blastocyst and cleavage-stage transfer. However, blastocyst transfer was associated with fewer patients having embryos frozen, as compared with cleavage-stage embryo transfer.[29]

When evaluating the outcomes of individual studies based on patient characteristics (such as age, number of previous failed attempts, ovarian response, and number and quality of embryos), there seems to be consistent evidence for higher pregnancy and live birth using fresh blastocyst transfer in good prognosis patients. However, implantation and pregnancy rates appear similar in women with at least two previous failed attempts, suggesting that the beneficial effect of blastocyst transfer may not be so prominent in patients with less good prognosis.[16]

The above findings highlight the concern that in vitro embryo survival may not necessarily equate to in-vivo survival, which significantly relies on the culture conditions. It has been proposed that by performing embryo transfer at the blastocyst stage, there is a theoretical risk of losing some embryos that do not survive in extended culture but that might have survived in vivo and resulted in a pregnancy if they had been transferred to the uterus earlier.[30]

The above concern has not been adequately addressed in studies involving human embryos. However, recent retrospective studies of patients with only one or two embryos have shown that blastocyst transfer was associated with similar or lower clinical pregnancy and live birth rates, and with higher transfer cancellation, compared to Day 3 transfer,[31] suggesting that in poorly responding patients with only few embryos available, transfer to the uterine environment at an earlier stage may be more beneficial than extended culture.

These observations are consistent with the results of a meta-analysis showing a higher incidence of cancelled transfers in unselected patients undergoing extended culture, but similar cancellation rates in good-prognosis patients.[32]

The questions that arise over the efficacy of blastocyst transfer are addressed by a retrospective study describing cumulative live birth rates after fresh and vitrified cleavage-stage vs. blastocyst-stage embryo transfer.[33] Blastocyst transfer was associated with higher live birth rates per started cycle and with fewer embryo transfers necessary until the first live birth. However, blastocyst transfer was also associated with fewer embryos available for cryopreservation and with higher transfer cancellation rates, compared to cleavage stage transfer. Importantly, the cumulative live birth rates were similar for cleavage-stage and blastocyst-stage transfers.

Despite the proposed advantages of blastocyst culture, several concerns have been expressed regarding the obstetric and perinatal outcomes of extended embryo culture. The topic has been subject to controversy for some time,[30,34] although it seems that the most recent data of children born after blastocyst transfer are reassuring.[35] (See further discussion in Chapter 11.)

The majority of early evidence suggests that blastocyst transfer is associated with a higher frequency of males compared with cleavage-stage embryo transfer or natural pregnancy.[16] A potential explanation of this observation may be that male embryos tend to develop faster, and embryologists inadvertently may preferentially select more developmentally advanced blastocysts for transfer. Nevertheless, the concept of altered sex ratio was challenged by recent data, showing that the chance of delivering a male baby was not increased by blastocyst-stage embryo transfer.[36]

8.3 The Morula Stage

The evolution of embryo culture systems has made possible the observation of all stages of human preimplantation development. However, the morphological examination and transfer of embryos is still almost exclusively performed at the cleavage (Day 2–3) or blastocyst (Day 5–6) stage. The morula stage seems neglected, possibly due to a more difficult morphology assessment, despite it involving crucial events that are decisive for future embryo development.

Indeed, recent knowledge obtained through live cell imaging technologies and cell biology studies have indicated that the morula is key stage for blastocyst development and the determination of the inner cell mass and the trophectoderm. In addition, time lapse monitoring has revealed that the process of compaction may be implicated in embryonic self-correction.[37]

There is a scarcity of RCTs, and a limited number of retrospective and observational studies, comparing Day 4 transfer with either Day 2/3 or Day 5/6. Therefore, current information on IVF outcomes after Day 4 transfer is very limited. A recent meta-analysis showed no difference in clinical pregnancy and ongoing pregnancy/live birth rates, transfer cancellation, and miscarriage rates, when comparing Day 4 with Day 2/3 and Day 5 embryo transfers. However, Day 4 transfer was associated with statistically significant lower preterm birth rates compared with Day 5 transfers (relative risk 0.19; 95% CI 0.05–0.67; $p = 0.01$), suggesting that the duration of embryo exposure to culture conditions is a topic that needs to be closely monitored in follow up longitudinal studies of offspring.[38]

In addition, the morula has been proposed as an alternative stage to perform embryo biopsy for PGT,[39] although its use by biopsy practitioners is currently very limited.

8.4 Embryos with Slow or Fast Development

It is recommended that embryos should follow a controlled cleavage rate: for human embryos this implies reaching the blastocyst stage on Day 5. It has been suggested that too slow or too fast embryo development has a negative impact on implantation rate and may be associated with a higher incidence of chromosomal abnormalities compared with normally developing embryos.[3]

However, there is evidence from retrospective studies that transfer of fast cleaving embryos with more than 10 cells on Day 3 had comparable clinical pregnancy and live birth rates compared with transfer of embryos at the 8-cell stage.

There is also more interest in the use of slowly developing embryos, forming the blastocyst in Day 7 of culture. Blastocysts are typically selected for transfer, biopsy, or cryopreservation on Days 5 and 6 of embryo culture. The practice of ending culture on Day 6 has been challenged recently by studies showing that Day 7 blastocysts, although slower compared to Days 5/6 blastocysts, can reach a top grade of morphology, and can result in a healthy live birth when transferred in a subsequent frozen replacement cycle, although they are associated with higher aneuploidy rates and lower live birth rates compared to Day 5 and 6 embryos.[40, 41]

The proportion of blastocyst utilization in those studies, expressed as a proportion of the total number of blastocysts cryopreserved, is approximately 65% for Day 5, 30% for Day 6, and 5% for Day 7.

Overall, it is proposed that culturing embryos until Day 7 increases the number of embryos for cryopreservation and biopsy, providing further opportunity for pregnancy for patients with only a few or low-quality blastocysts.[40, 41]

To this end, it has also been proposed that Day 6 morulae should be considered for biopsy in women <40 years old undergoing PGT for aneuploidy (PGT-A) because they are associated with acceptable, albeit reduced, euploidy and implantation rates.[42]

8.5 Conclusions

The timing and duration of embryo culture are crucial for embryo viability and IVF success. The evolution of suitable culture media able to sustain all stages of preimplantation embryo development has increased the popularity of blastocyst culture. Blastocyst culture seems to have some competitive advantages over cleavage-stage transfer, including improved selection and promotion of eSET, synchronization with the uterine environment, trophectoderm biopsy, cryopreservation efficiency, and monitoring of OHSS. Blastocyst transfer seems to be associated with higher pregnancy and live birth rates compared to cleavage-stage transfer, although this effect is more pronounced in good prognosis patients with many embryos. On the other hand, cleavage-stage transfer still has a place, and may be even recommended in some cases, for poor prognosis patients, such as women with poor ovarian response, in whom blastocyst culture results in high transfer cancellation rates. It must be noted that although blastocyst transfer may reduce the time needed time to achieve a live birth, it does not increase cumulative live birth rates compared to cleavage-stage transfer. Recent data on the health of children born are reassuring, and suggest that perinatal outcomes are similar after cleavage-stage and blastocyst transfer.

References

1. Niakan KK, Han J, Pedersen RA, Simon C, Pera RA. Human pre-implantation embryo development. *Development*. 2012;139:829–841.

2. Van Royen E, Mangelschots K, De Neubourg D, et al. Characterization of a top quality embryo, a step towards single-embryo transfer. *Hum Reprod*. 1999;14: 2345–2349.

3. Alpha Scientists in Reproductive Medicine and ESHRE Special Interest Group of Embryology. The Istanbul consensus workshop on embryo assessment: proceedings of an expert meeting. *Hum Reprod*. 2011;26:1270–1283.

4. Magli MC, Gianaroli L, Ferraretti AP, Lappi M, Ruberti A, Farfalli V. Embryo morphology and development are dependent on the chromosomal complement. *Fertil Steril*. 2007;87:534–541.

5. Whitten WK. Culture of tubal mouse ova. *Nature*. 1956;177:96.

6. McLaren A, Biggers JD. Successful development and birth of mice cultivated in vitro as early as early embryos. *Nature*. 1958;182:877–878.

7. Quinn P. Culture systems: Sequential. In: Smith GD, Swain JE, Pool TB. (eds) *Methods in Molecular Biology*, 912. Totawa, NJ: Humana Press; 2012: 211–230.

8. Gardner DK, Lane M. Culture and selection of viable blastocysts: a feasible proposition for human IVF? *Hum Reprod Update*. 1997;3: 367–382.

9. Machtinger R, Racowsky C. Culture systems: Single step. In: Smith GD, Swain JE, Pool TB. (eds) *Methods in Molecular Biology*, 912. Totawa, NJ: Humana Press;2012:199–209.

10. Sfontouris IA, Martins WP, Nastri CO, Viana IG, et al. Blastocyst culture using single versus sequential media in clinical IVF: a systematic review and meta-analysis of randomized controlled trials. *J Assist Reprod Genet*. 2016;33: 1261–1272.

11. Bourdon, M, Pocate-Cheriet K, Finet de Bantel A, et al. Day 5 versus Day 6 blastocyst transfers: a systematic review and meta-analysis of clinical outcomes. *Hum Reprod*. 2019;34:1948–1964.

12. Tannus S, Cohen Y, Henderson S, et al. Fresh transfer of Day 5 slow-growing embryos versus deferred transfer of vitrified, fully expanded Day 6 blastocysts: which is the optimal approach? *Hum Reprod*. 2019;34:44–51.

13. Arce JC, Ziebe S, Lundin K, Janssens R, Helmgaard L, Sørensen P. Interobserver agreement and intraobserver reproducibility of embryo quality assessments. *Hum Reprod*. 2006;21:2141–2148.

14. Rijnders PM, Jansen CA. The predictive value of day 3 embryo morphology regarding blastocyst formation, pregnancy and implantation rate after day 5 transfer following in-vitro fertilization or intracytoplasmic sperm injection. *Hum Reprod*. 1998;13: 2869–2873.

15. Minasi MG, Colasante A, Riccio T, et al. Correlation between aneuploidy, standard morphology evaluation and morphokinetic development in 1730 biopsied blastocysts: a consecutive case series study. *Hum Reprod*. 2016;31: 2245–2254.

16. Practice Committee of the American Society for Reproductive Medicine. Blastocyst culture and transfer in clinically assisted reproduction: a committee opinion. *Fertil Steril*. 2018;110: 1246–1252.

17. Berntsen S, Soderstrom-Anttila V, Wennerholm UB, et al. The health of children conceived by ART: 'the chicken or the egg?'. *Hum Reprod Update*. 2019; 25: 137–158.

18. ESHRE PGT Consortium and SIG-Embryology Biopsy Working Group, Kokkali G, Coticchio G, Bronet F, Celebi C, Cimadomo D, Goossens V, Liss J, Nunes S, Sfontouris I, Vermeulen N, Zakharova E, De Rycke M. *Hum Reprod Open*. 2020; 29: 2020(3).

19. Scott RT, Jr, Upham KM, Forman EJ, Zhao T, Treff NR. Cleavage-stage biopsy significantly impairs human embryonic implantation potential while blastocyst biopsy does not: a randomized and paired clinical trial. *Fertil Steril*. 2013;100: 624–630.

20. Van de Velde H, De Vos A, Sermon K, et al. Embryo implantation after biopsy of one or two cells from cleavage-stage embryos with a view to preimplantation genetic diagnosis. *Prenat Diagn*. 2000;20: 1030–1037.

21. Geraedts J, Sermon K. Preimplantation genetic screening 2.0: the theory. *Mol Hum Reprod*. 2016;22:839–844.

22. Glujovsky D, Farquhar C, Quinteiro Retamar AM, Alvarez Sedo CR, Blake D. Cleavage stage versus blastocyst stage embryo

transfer in assisted reproductive technology. *Cochrane Database Syst Rev.* 2016;(6):CD002118. doi: 10.1002/14651858.CD002118. pub5.

23. Cobo A, de los Santos MJ, Castello D, Gamiz P, Campos P, Remohi J. Outcomes of vitrified early cleavage-stage and blastocyst-stage embryos in a cryopreservation program: evaluation of 3,150 warming cycles. *Fertil Steril.* 2012;98: 1138–1146 e1.

24. Fernandez-Shaw S, Cercas R, Brana C, Villas C, Pons I. Ongoing and cumulative pregnancy rate after cleavage-stage versus blastocyst-stage embryo transfer using vitrification for cryopreservation: impact of age on the results. *J Assist Reprod Genet.* 2015;32: 177–184.

25. Morbeck DE. Blastocyst culture in the Era of PGS and FreezeAlls: Is a 'C' a failing grade? *Human Reprod Open.* 2017;2017:hox017.

26. Devroey P, Polyzos NP, Blockeel C. An OHSS-free clinic by segmentation of IVF treatment. *Human Reprod.* 2011;26: 2593–2597.

27. Nastri CO, Teixeira DM, Moroni RM, Leitao VM, Martins WP. Ovarian hyperstimulation syndrome: pathophysiology, staging, prediction and prevention. *Ultrasound Obstet Gynecol.* 2015;45:377–393.

28. Lainas G, Kolibianakis E, Sfontouris I, et al. Outpatient management of severe early OHSS by administration of GnRH antagonist in the luteal phase: an observational cohort study. *Reprod Biol Endocrinol.* 2012;10:69.

29. Martins WP, Nastri CO, Rienzi L, van der Poel SZ, Gracia C, Racowsky C. Blastocyst vs cleavage-stage embryo transfer: systematic review and meta-analysis of reproductive outcomes. *Ultrasound Obstet Gynecol.* 2017;49: 583–591.

30. Maheshwari A, Hamilton M, Bhattacharya S. Should we be promoting embryo transfer at blastocyst stage? *Reprod Biomed Online.* 2016;32:142–146.

31. Xiao JS, Healey M, Talmor A, Vollenhoven B. When only one embryo is available, is it better to transfer on Day 3 or to grow on? *Reprod BioMedicine Online.* 2019;39: 916–923.

32. Papanikolaou EG, Kolibianakis EM, Tournaye H, et al. Live birth rates after transfer of equal number of blastocysts or cleavage-stage embryos in IVF. A systematic review and meta-analysis. *Human Reprod.* 2007;23: 91–99.

33. De Vos A, Van Landuyt L, Santos-Ribeiro S, et al. Cumulative live birth rates after fresh and vitrified cleavage-stage versus blastocyst-stage embryo transfer in the first treatment cycle. *Hum Reprod.* 2016;31: 2442–2449.

34. Gardner DK. The impact of physiological oxygen during culture, and vitrification for cryopreservation, on the outcome of extended culture in human IVF. *Reprod Biomed Online.* 2016;32: 137–141.

35. Marconi N, Raja EA, Bhattacharya S, Maheshwari A. Perinatal outcomes in singleton live births after fresh blastocyst-stage embryo transfer: a retrospective analysis of 67 147 IVF/ICSI cycles. *Hum Reprod.* 2019;34:1716–1725.

36. Busnelli A, Dallagiovanna C, Reschini M, Paffoni A, Fedele L, Somigliana E. Risk factors for monozygotic twinning after in vitro fertilization: a systematic review and meta-analysis. *Fertil Steril.* 2019;111: 302–317.

37. Coticchio G, Lagalla C, Sturmey R, Pennetta F, Borini A. The enigmatic morula: mechanisms of development, cell fate determination, self-correction and implications for ART. *Hum Reprod Update.* 2019;25: 422–438.

38. Simopoulou M, Sfakianoudis K, Tsioulou P, et al. Should the flexibility enabled by performing a day-4 embryo transfer remain a valid option in the IVF laboratory? A systematic review and network meta-analysis. *J Assist Reprod Genet.* 2019;36:1049–1061.

39. Zakharova EE, Zaletova VV, Krivokharchenko AS. Biopsy of human morula-stage embryos: outcome of 215 IVF/ICSI cycles with PGS. *PLoS One* 2014;9: e106433.

40. Hammond ER, Cree LM, Morbeck DE. Should extended blastocyst culture include Day 7? *Human Reprod.* 2018;33:991–997.

41. Hernandez-Nieto C, Lee JA, Slifkin R, Sandler B, Copperman AB, Flisser E. What is the reproductive potential of day 7 euploid embryos? *Human Reprod.* 2019;34:1697–1706.

42. Irani M, Zaninovic N, Canon C, et al. A rationale for biopsying embryos reaching the morula stage on Day 6 in women undergoing preimplantation genetic testing for aneuploidy. *Human Reprod.* 2018;33:935–941.

Chapter

9

Time-Lapse Technology
Theoretical and Practical Aspects

Kirstine Kirkegaard and Thomas Freour

9.1 Introduction

Optimal culture conditions and reliable embryo selection are two fundamental laboratory aspects of successful IVF treatment, with the overall aim being to obtain a healthy singleton pregnancy in the shortest possible time. This chapter will cover the use of time-lapse technology (TLT) for continuous morphological evaluation of the embryo within an undisturbed culture. The first part will address the evidence for improving clinical outcome and the development of selection models; the second part will cover the practical aspects of the use and implementation of TLT.

9.2 Evidence-Based Use of Time-Lapse Technology

9.2.1 Time-Lapse vs. Morphological Selection

As there is a well-documented correlation between embryo morphology at given time points and developmental competence, the quality and viability of preimplantation embryos are traditionally evaluated by microscopic inspection at a few, well-defined discrete time points. Morphological grading is simple, relatively easy to learn, and cost-effective. The method, however, has several limitations. As the collected information has been limited to a few time points, it gives an incomplete picture of the dynamic embryo development. Several transient aspects of potential importance, such as number of pronuclei, are easily missed. Furthermore, morphological scoring is relatively subjective, as demonstrated by large inter- as well as intra-observer variability. This variability has implications for the decision to transfer, cryopreserve, or discard the embryos, with a rather low reproducibility. Finally, the standard morphological evaluation requires that embryos are removed from the incubator for assessment, thereby exposing the embryos to changes in temperature, humidity, and gas composition that may be potentially harmful.

There are two obvious benefits to TLT that may be translated into improved clinical outcome: Improved culture conditions and improved embryo selection. Firstly, images for embryo assessment are obtained without removing embryos from the incubator. Although TLT necessitates periodical light exposure, use of moving devices, and magnetic fields, which may all be of potential harm to the embryos, continuous culture made possible by TLT eliminates the exposure of embryos to the stress of mechanical moving and changes in temperature, humidity, and gas composition and is therefore most likely to improve culture conditions.

Secondly, TLT captures the dynamics of embryo development more extensively. In addition to a more precise registration of events, such as timing of cellular divisions until compaction, timing of the morula stage, formation of the blastocoel, blastocyst expansion, and – in some cases – collapse and reformation and eventually hatching, temporary events missed by static evaluation are easily recorded by TLT. Examples that have all been evaluated in several publications are time for formation of the male pronucleus, extrusion of the second polar body followed by formation of the male and female pronuclei, and syngamy/abuttal and disappearance of the pronuclei. From the time points recorded, duration of cellular stages can be calculated and deviations from normal development can be observed, e.g., extremely short duration of the first division cycle (the 2-cell stage), referred to as a direct cleavage from one to three cells. This information may be used to improve embryo selection. Numerous observational studies have been published demonstrating higher implantation rates using a diversity of time-lapse markers and selection models. There are, however, very few studies that have validated their findings in independent populations, and even fewer randomized trials. Given the scope of the present chapter, only prospective studies will be discussed.

In principle, prospective studies can be designed to evaluate the effect of uninterrupted culture, improved embryo selection, or both. Only very few studies have evaluated the isolated effect. Most studies have evaluated the combined effect of uninterrupted culture and time-lapse selection. A recent Cochrane meta-analysis has summarized the evidence from published RCTs (Armstrong et al., 2019).

Six randomized trials have compared culture in a standard incubator to a time-lapse incubator. All six trials were conducted using an integrated device. Two studies were performed randomizing oocytes rather than patients, and evaluated embryo development on day 3 as primary endpoint, where no difference was found. The evidence from these two trials is low quality, and they were excluded from a recent Cochrane analysis. The remaining four studies were, however, included in the Cochrane analysis (Armstrong et al., 2019). The designs in these four studies were heterogenous, in particular day of embryo transfer was different in all four studies. Three studies provided data on ongoing pregnancy or live births. Based on a meta-analysis of these three studies (3 RCTs, $N = 826$), there is no evidence for any difference between uninterrupted culture and standard incubation (OR 0.91, 95% CI 0.67–1.23).

Only two randomized studies have evaluated the isolated effect of time-lapse selection vs. standard morphological selection under identical culture conditions. One study evaluated ongoing pregnancy following day 3 single embryo transfer with TLT vs. day 5 single embryo transfer with or without adjunctive TLT (Kaser et al., 2017). The study found a nonsignificant higher clinical pregnancy rates in the D5 arm without TLT (OR 0.76 (0.34–1.66), 0.76 (0.34–1.66), and 1.00 (referent) for D3 + TLT, D5 + TLT, and D5 standard evaluation alone, respectively). The authors concluded that although the study was not powered (due to premature termination by the sponsor, Eeva) the higher clinical pregnancy rate in the D5 standard evaluation alone arm, suggested that use of early time-lapse markers may not improve embryo selection. The second randomized study reported clinical pregnancy rates and found no difference between TLT and standard evaluation (Goodman et al., 2016).

Three studies were included in the meta-analysis on clinical pregnancy and live birth evaluating the combination of continued culture and selection using TLT. Based on a meta-analysis of these studies (3 RCTs, $N = 826$), no difference between TLT and standard evaluation was found between interventions in rates of live birth (OR 1.12, 95% CI 0.92–1.36, 3 RCTs, $N = 1617$). The authors stress that there was a high risk of bias in the included studies and the high level of heterogeneity in study design. Of particular importance is that randomization was broken in the largest of the studies, as some of the patients received the intervention based on request rather than randomization.

Overall, the Cochrane review concludes that there is insufficient good-quality evidence of differences in live birth or ongoing pregnancy or clinical pregnancy to choose between TLT, with or without embryo selection software, and conventional incubation. In contrast, another meta-analysis including five RCTS concludes that TLT with the prospective use of a morphokinetic algorithm for selection of embryos improves overall clinical outcome (Pribenszky et al., 2017). Concerns were, however, raised based on inconsistency of inclusion and exclusion of studies, data analysis, classification of bias and heterogeneity, and conflict of interest, as all authors were employees of a company supplying time-lapse incubators.

Since the first commercial time-lapse instruments were introduced 10 years ago, several instruments have become available, and TLT and continuous culture are implemented in large numbers. Clinical RCTs are time-consuming, but without question the gold standard of evidence-based medicine. Based on the available low-quality evidence, it seems reasonable to comply with the recommendation of ESHRE's recent guideline (2020) that more RCTs with adequate design and sufficient power be conducted, reporting on live births and perinatal outcomes, in order to firmly establish a putative beneficial effect of TLT.

9.2.2 Time-Lapse Prediction Models

A crucial part of implementing time-lapse in the laboratory is to decide on which parameters to annotate and evaluate. Some instruments offer automated annotation, and predefined selection models. Ideally, each clinic should evaluate their own data in order to develop an in-house algorithm or selection strategy

Table 9.1 Examples of parameters used in different time-lapse models

Study	$n_{embryos}$	Parameters
Meseguer et al., 2011	$n = 247$	Inclusion: t5 (48.8–56.6 h), t4–t3(<0.76 h), t3–t2/cc2 (<11.9 h). Exclusion: direct cleavage, multinucleation, uneven blastomeres (2-cell)
Azzarello et al., 2012	$n = 159$	Pronuclear breakdown
Aguilar et al., 2014	$n = 899$	Extrusion 2nd polar body, pronuclear appearance to fading and pronuclear fading
Athayde Wirka et al., 2014	$n = 122$	Abnormal syngamy, abnormal first cytokinesis, abnormal cleavage, or chaotic cleavage
VerMilyea et al., 2014	$n = 331$	High P2 9.33–11.45 h; P3 0–1.73 h. Medium P2 9.33–12.65 h; P3 0–4 h
Basile et al., 2015	$n = 1664$	t3 (34–40 h), t3–t2 (9–12 h), and t5 (45–55h). Exclusion: direct cleavage, multinucleation 4-cell stage, uneven blastomeres (2-cell)
Liu et al., 2015	$n = 270$	Conventional morphology, abnormal cleavage, t5, 3-cell stage
Adamson et al., 2016	$n = 319$	P2 9.33–11.45 h and P3 0–1.73 h. Exclusion: direct cleavage
Goodman et al., 2016 (RCT)	$n = 235$	Negative points: cc2 <5 h (−1), presence of multinucleation (−0.5), presence of irregular division (−0.5). Positive points: t5 45.8–57.0 HPI (+1), s2 0.0–0.1 h (+1), s3 1.4–7.0 h (+1), tSB <100 HPI (+1).
Yang et al., 2018 (RCT)	$n = 600$	Abnormal cleavage
Petersen et al., 2018	$n = 11218$	t3–tPNf, t5–t3/t3–t2
Fishel et al., 2018	$n = 781$	Start blastulation, duration of blastulation
Kovacs et al., 2019 (RCT)	$n = 161$	cc1, cc2, 1st cytokinesis, S2, t5, fragmentation, vacuolization

cc1: t2–t0
cc2/ P2: t3–t2
s2/P3: t4–t3
HPI: hours post insemination/injection
t2, t3, t4. . . .: Time to division to 2, 3, 4. . . blastomeres, respectively
cc1, cc2, cc3. . . : duration of cell cycle 1, 2, 3 (also called P1, P2, P3..)
s2, s3: synchronization of cell cycles 2, 3,
tPNF: time to pronuclear fading

designed for their particular patient population and culture conditions. This is, however, very time-consuming and requires a large dataset. Therefore, clinics often refer to the literature for guidance. ESHRE recommendations for practical use of TLT have recently been published (2020).

A large amount of observational studies has suggested different parameters and time-intervals. A non-exhaustive overview is presented in Table 9.1. The most thoroughly tested model is the hierarchical model presented by Meseguer et al. in 2011 (Meseguer et al., 2011), which has been tested in a RCT and subsequently refined using large datasets. The model ranks embryos based on a combination of de-selection (poor morphology, direct cleavage from 1 to 3 cells, uneven blastomere size at 2-cell stage, and multinucleation at 4-cell stage) and selection based on timings (t5 (48.8–56.6 hours), t4–t3 (<0.76 hours), t3–t2/cc2 (<11.9 hours). When tested in an RCT ($n = 856$), an OR of 1.23 (1.06–1.43) in favor of the study group for the primary outcome of ongoing pregnancy rate along was reported. The embryos in the study group were cultured in a standard incubator, therefore the individual contribution of the effect of TL selection cannot be separated from the effect of different incubators. In addition, the randomization was broken, as some of the patients were assigned to TLT by request after randomization, introducing potential bias. Finally, nearly half of the patients received embryos from oocyte donors, which limits the external validity. Another prediction model tested in several studies is the model suggested by Eeva, where embryos are ranked in high/low categories based on early time intervals (Table 9.1; VerMilyea, Adamson). The model has been tested (with modifications) in one RCTs (Kaser et al., 2017), where no difference was found, however the study was terminated early.

All of the models have proved difficult to transfer from one clinical setting to another. A plausible explanation is that timing of development is influenced by a variety of patient- and treatment-related factors, such as oxygen tension, fertilization method, culture media, smoking, age, baseline androgen levels, and type of gonadotropin used for stimulation (ESHRE 2020). Consequently, a prediction model that is developed from one dataset will most likely perform well only on the dataset it was developed from, or on datasets from similar clinical conditions, in particular if the dataset is small and the clinical characteristics narrow. An important limitation of the majority of studies is, therefore, that they have not been validated on independent datasets, which limits the transferability. Furthermore, several of the observational studies have not taken into account that timing of embryo development not only reflects viability, but is heavily influenced by patient characteristics. Consequently, several observational studies tend to overestimate the predictive power of the identified parameters.

Another important consideration when developing prediction models is to weight sensitivity against specificity. Several of the early models defined very narrow time intervals for optimal division to achieve high specificity at the expense of a low sensitivity. As they were developed on small datasets, this subsequently limited transferability and introduced a high risk of discarding viable embryos if transferred uncritically. On the other hand, using too broad intervals lowers the value of the algorithm, as no real ranking is performed. In general, a model that aims at de-selecting embryos with low viability would be expected to be more transferable to other settings than a model based on narrow intervals for optimal division. Recently, an algorithm based on large datasets of heterogeneous origin has been developed, which theoretically should be applicable to different culture conditions and patient-groups (Petersen et al., 2016). The algorithm has not been tested in randomized studies.

9.2.3 Time-Lapse and Computer Assisted Technology/Machine Learning

TLT generates a large amount of images. Manual evaluation of all the available information is unattainable in daily practice and potentially valuable information is therefore lost; consequently, time-lapse data are currently underutilized in clinical decision making. Furthermore, traditional statistical methods often prove insufficient for the large amount of data generated. The rapidly developing field of artificial intelligence (AI) may prove to be the missing link that will utilize the full potential of the technology in daily clinic. Overall, AI refers to various methods where machines can learn to perform intelligent tasks like humans, allowing for automation of various procedures, or better than humans, resulting in improved outcome. In particular, deep learning that is part of a broader family of machine learning methods based on artificial neural networks has been applied for analysis of imaging in medicine. A deep learning process can directly analyze all the time-lapse images and correlate to outcome, without the need for manual annotation parameters. The obvious benefit lies in the potential for full automation, use of all available information instead of a few time-points, and objectiveness. The technology is still in its infancy, but several projects are being undertaken to establish the appropriate use. In a recent publication, the technology has been used to classify embryos and predict fetal heart beat (Tran et al., 2019). With an impressing area under the curve (AUC) of the method to predict pregnancy on the dataset of 0.93 (95% CI 0.92–0.94), full reproducibility, and transferability, the approach is extremely promising. Apart from the automation and objectivity, it may render the need for developing prediction models based on few parameters redundant.

9.3 Practical Aspects of TLT Clinical Use

Although high-quality evidence remains to be presented, the combined benefit of TLT on embryo culture conditions and embryo quality evaluation is now widely accepted, and the technique is therefore increasingly being implemented into clinical practice. However, use of TLT in the IVF laboratory is not unproblematic for either staff or lab organization, and raises some technical and practical issues. Use of TLT necessitates definition of novel morphokinetic parameters that can be used for decision making, as well as the definition of a new workflow in the laboratory.

9.3.1 Types and Characteristics of TLT devices

9.3.1.1 Single vs. Combined Embryo Culture

TLT requires embryos to be cultured individually in order to annotate morphokinetic features and follow the development of each embryo separately. With the exception of the PrimoVision® TLT system, where embryos are only separated from each other by a very small wall, all TLT systems available on the market use specifically designed culture dishes providing individual micro-wells for each embryo. Although embryos are cultured in individual micro-wells in most cases, some dishes allow them to be covered by a single large drop of culture medium, theoretically allowing inter-embryo contact while other dishes consist of completely separated individual drops of culture medium without contact with other wells. There is no evidence to date to suggest the superiority of one design vs. the other in terms of embryo development. From a handling point of view, the various types of dishes do not differ significantly from each other, and all require specific training and attention.

9.3.1.2 Image Acquisition

Image acquisition is critical for proper and relevant analysis of embryo development. In this respect, TLT devices should not only provide excellent images in terms of definition, but the frequency of image acquisition should allow continuous monitoring without impairing embryo development and/or overload computer storage capacity.

TLT devices have various specifications, some being adjustable by the user. The first aspect of image acquisition concerns the number of focal planes. This parameter is important for the evaluation of the whole embryo in three dimensions, especially at late developmental stages (blastocyst). All TLT devices allow the acquisition of several focal planes (3–17). This parameter is fixed in some devices and can be adjusted in others. There are no specific guidelines on the ideal number of focal planes that should be used, and each TLT user may decide the optimal setting from their own clinical experience.

The second aspect concerns the time interval between image acquisitions. This parameter is obviously important for the evaluation of embryo development in order to observe all cellular events, including fugitive and rapid ones. Once again, this parameter is fixed in some devices and can be adjusted in others. Overall, this time interval ranges between 5 and 60 min. Short time intervals allow better observation of embryo development, but very few cellular events occur in less than 10 or even 20 minutes, thus questioning the relevance of extremely short time intervals. At present, there are no specific guidelines on the ideal time interval between image acquisitions.

The type and duration of embryo light exposure varies between TLT devices, but all offer extremely short illumination and use LED with precise wave length outside the toxic spectrum. This cannot be adjusted and should not be considered as an issue when considering TLT (Rong et al., 2014). Finally, the type of camera and the optical method used for image acquisition also differ among TLT devices. While most TLT devices use brightfield microscopy (with or without Hoffman modulation), which is the method of choice in IVF laboratories, some propose darkfield microscopy or oblique illumination. The number of megapixels of the camera (and quality of the screen where images are displayed) obviously determines image quality, but in general, all TLT devices offer good image resolution.

9.3.1.3 Integrated vs. Nonintegrated Systems

As far as the authors are aware, only one TLT system currently available on the market is a nonintegrated system, i.e., placed in a conventional incubator (PrimoVision®). All other systems are fully integrated, combining incubation chamber and image acquisition in a global device. Although nonintegrated TLT systems also provide the benefit of continuous embryo monitoring with repeated image acquisition, the quality of culture conditions will depend on the frequency of door openings and the recovery of temperature and gas atmosphere. It can be speculated that nonintegrated TLT systems offer less stable and precise embryo culture conditions than integrated TLT systems. However, any clinical superiority of integrated TLT systems over nonintegrated TLT systems is not yet reported in the literature.

9.3.1.4 Gas

The superiority of low oxygen tension over ambient oxygen in terms of embryo development in vitro and IVF clinical outcome has been demonstrated over the last two decades. All TLT devices currently available on the market offer the possibility of performing embryo culture under low oxygen tension. Oxygen concentration can even be precisely adjusted in order to suit the specific operative procedures of the IVF laboratory. Some TLT devices include an integrated gas mixer, allowing the connection to the nitrogen and CO_2 supply pipes. However, some other TLT devices require the use of premixed gas bottles. This aspect should be considered when investing in TLT systems in order to avoid unnecessary additional gas handling and costs.

9.3.2 Operating and Using TLT

9.3.2.1 Dish Preparation and Handling

All TLT systems require the use of specific embryo culture dishes for proper image acquisition. After initial training of all operators by the supplier and/or the local referent, specific operating procedures must be set up and followed by the whole staff in order to ensure safe and correct handling of these dishes. For instance, to ensure optimal image acquisition the introduction of air bubbles in embryo culture wells must be avoided and embryos need to be properly loaded, generally with micro-tips, right in the center of the image acquisition area and at the bottom of the well.

9.3.2.2 TLT for Embryo Quality Assessment

Embryo development can be followed live and evaluated on the TLT device itself or on a remote computer. It can also be observed later on recorded files.

Importantly, guidelines have been published in order to standardize embryo morphokinetic annotation in order to limit interoperator variability, within and across centers (Ciray et al., 2014).

TLT offers several advantages over conventional morphology assessment in terms of embryo quality assessment. Practically, the recording of all images and videos allows in depth analysis of cellular events, with precise measurement of timings, and facilitates staff discussion and shared decisions. TLT is of particular interest at the blastocyst stage, when embryo development is rapidly changing, and evaluations can be problematic due to contractions, excluded cells, and fragments.

From a practical point of view, all TLT systems are associated with software installed on a computer, where all pictures/videos are saved in real time, allowing remote and/or delayed embryo annotation. The observation of embryo development is feasible with TLT software, either image by image, or as a video, and the operator's role is to identify and record the time points when relevant embryo developmental events occur. Most software can be customized by the user, either to annotate only a few morphokinetic parameters considered to be relevant or to annotate an extensive list of all cellular events and morphological features.

Recently, some TLT software implemented a semiautomated identification of main cleavage events, aimed at saving operator's time and improving annotation workflow. In practice, the operator's attention is directed to time periods where these cellular events often occur, reducing the time spent playing the video between these events. It is likely that these automated systems will develop and improve, probably leading to fully automated annotation systems in the near future.

9.3.3 TLT Use in Preimplantation Genetic Testing Cycles

Preimplantation genetic testing for aneuploidy (PGT-A), has developed extensively over recent years, with a clear shift from day 3 embryo biopsy to trophectoderm biopsy, allowing more accurate evaluation of embryo chromosomal status and improved clinical outcome (Treff & Zimmerman, 2017). From a practical and organizational point of view, TLT can be considered to be beneficial to PGT-A program in two ways.

First, morphokinetic parameters obtained with TLT have been shown to be associated with embryo ploidy status (reviewed in Reignier et al., 2018). However, although most studies found significant differences in morphokinetic parameters between euploid and aneuploid embryos, none demonstrated that TLT should be considered as a relevant alternative for PGT-A (Reignier ct al., 2018; Zaninovic et al., 2017). Interestingly, the observation of direct uneven cleavages at early stages with TLT was associated in most studies with very low implantation rate or even absence of implantation in the case of direct cleavage from zygote to 3-cell embryo (Rubio et al., 2012; Zhan et al., 2016). This drop in implantation despite acceptable morphology is believed to be associated with embryo aneuploidy and TLT may thereby help to identify aneuploid embryos without PGT-A in this specific case (Zhan et al., 2016). Furthermore, morphokinetic analysis has been shown to help in selecting the embryo with the highest implantation potential among those diagnosed as euploid after PGT-A (Rocafort et al., 2018).

Second, performing trophectoderm biopsy at the blastocyst stage has raised the issue of how to spot the best moment for biopsy. As the blastocyst is a very dynamic stage, with heterogeneous developmental speed among embryos of the same cohort, the optimal time to perform blastocyst biopsy will differ for each embryo. TLT avoids taking out embryos of the incubator to determine development stage, and allows precise and live evaluation of blastocyst expansion and trophectoderm herniation, making it a useful tool for daily PGT-A practice in the IVF laboratory.

9.3.4 TLT as a Training/Teaching Tool

Teaching clinical embryology to beginners and maintaining competence in experienced embryologists has long been a difficult task for University teachers and IVF lab supervisors, especially because of the need to use static images of embryos or organize training in the lab at specific time points when dishes are taken out of the incubators to assess embryo quality.

In this respect, TLT provides a revolutionary tool for teaching clinical embryology. An extremely high number of images are available with TLT, allowing image and video libraries with both normal and abnormal developmental events. These libraries can be used as an educational support tool available at any time, and also as an internal quality control tool to ascertain lab staff's competence.

Unfortunately, only a few independent TLT training programs are available as yet, and most training is conducted by TLT suppliers. These training programs are essential to provide and maintain technical and data interpretation skills.

9.3.5 Management of IVF Staff and Work-Flow

The decision to implement TLT in the IVF lab should be followed by reflections and setting up of protocols on how to apply the technology efficiently, both from a human resource and a workflow perspective. Indeed, TLT implementation will have several consequences on IVF lab workflow, but provides a great opportunity to optimize procedures and organization.

9.3.5.1 Rethinking IVF Lab Work-Flow with TLT

Contrary to conventional incubation which requires microscopic evaluation of embryos at fixed timepoints, TLT allows recording of embryos 24/7, thus giving the opportunity to review and score embryo development at any time, and when it is more convenient for the staff. So, at times during the day when the workload for staff is high, the risk of adverse events can be minimized with the use of TLT and reorganizing of embryo evaluations to less busy periods of time in the day. Embryo development can also be evaluated remotely via an internet secure connection.

It is important to note that many IVF labs use TLT in parallel with conventional incubators and static grading. In this respect, it is important that both strategies are integrated and complementary, and do not disrupt each other.

9.3.5.2 Staff Management and Quality Control Policy

As requested in all quality control policies, IVF staff needs to write and use scrupulously its own standard operating procedures (SOPs) for TLT clinical use. These SOPs should describe both technical (how to run the machine) and biological aspects (how to use clinically the data generated by TLT).

Conventional embryo morphology grading suffers from intra- and inter-observer variability, potentially impairing its clinical relevance. Although TLT allows a more precise and reproducible evaluation of embryo quality (Martínez, et al., 2018; Martinez-Granados et al., 2017; Sundvall et al., 2013), quality controls should be implemented to ensure that morphokinetic annotation remains stable for all participants and over time. This is particularly true for cellular events occurring progressively, such as pronuclear formation, morula compaction, or blastocyst expansion, whose evaluation is more difficult to standardize, thus requiring a clear and consensual definition. Altogether, IVF staff should be regularly trained in order to ensure proper use of the machine, very limited inter-operator variation for annotation, and consistent decision-making process. In this respect, the staff should participate in a regular internal quality control program. Although its frequency and composition can vary between centres, participation should be mandatory for the whole staff, and acceptable performance thresholds should be clearly defined by supervisors, so that operators with insufficient performance can be rapidly detected and specifically trained. Some countries have already implemented similar external quality controls, and it can be anticipated that commercial external quality controls specifically devoted to TLT will soon be available on the market. TLT could also be considered in the future as a valuable tool for quality control of IVF protocols (Kovacic et al., 2018) and consumables, such as culture media (Ferrick et al., 2019).

9.4 Summary

TLT potentially improves embryo culture conditions and embryo quality evaluation, but its clinical usefulness and its superiority over conventional morphological grading still remains debated. Presently, there is insufficient good-quality evidence that demonstrates differences in live birth or ongoing pregnancy or clinical pregnancy between TLT and conventional incubation and selection. Accordingly, the recent recommendation of ESHRE is that more RCTs with adequate design and sufficient power should be conducted in order to firmly establish a putative beneficial effect of TLT.

The development of new prediction models and the combined use of AI technologies might move things forward in the near future. Knowing the characteristics of TLT devices and how to operate them and integrate them in the lab's work-flow is of utmost importance when considering its implementation, as it has several implications for daily practice and staff management.

References

Adamson GD, Abusief ME, Palao L, Witmer J, Palao LM, Gvakharia M. Improved implantation rates of day 3 embryo transfers with the use of an automated time-lapse–enabled test to aid in embryo selection. *Fert Ster.* 2016;105:369–375. e366.

Aguilar J, Motato Y, Escriba MJ, Ojeda M, Munoz E, Meseguer M. The human first cell cycle: impact on implantation. *Reprod Biomed Online.* 2014;28:475–484.

Athayde Wirka K, Chen AA, Conaghan J, et al. Atypical embryo phenotypes identified by time-lapse microscopy: high prevalence and association with embryo development. *Fert Ster.* 2014;101: 1637–1648. e5.

Armstrong S, Bhide P, Jordan V, Pacey A, Marjoribanks J, Farquhar C. Time-lapse systems for embryo incubation and assessment in assisted reproduction. *Cochrane Database Syst Rev.* 2019(5):Cd011320.

Azzarello A, Hoest T, Mikkelsen AL. 2012. The impact of pronuclei morphology and dynamicity on live birth outcome after time-lapse culture. *Human Reprod.* 2012;27: 2649–2657.

Basile N, Vime P, Florensa M, et al. 2015. The use of morphokinetics as a predictor of implantation: a multicentric study to define and validate an algorithm for embryo selection. *Human Reprod.* 30:276–283.

Ciray HN, Campbell A, Agerholm IE, et al. Proposed guidelines on the nomenclature and annotation of dynamic human embryo monitoring by a time-lapse user group. *Human Reprod.* 2014;29:2650–2660.

ESHRE Working group on Time-Lapse Technology. Good practice recommendations for the use of time-lapse technology. *Human Reprod Open.* 2020(2); 2020: hoaa008.

Ferrick L, Lee YSL, Gardner DK. Reducing time to pregnancy and facilitating the birth of healthy children through functional analysis of embryo physiology. *Biol Reprod.* 2019;101:1124–1139.

Fishel S, Campbell A, Montgomery S, et al. Time-lapse imaging algorithms rank human preimplantation embryos according to the probability of live birth. *Reprod Biomed Online.* 2018;37:304–313.

Goodman LR, Goldberg J, Falcone T, Austin C, Desai N. Does the addition of time-lapse morphokinetics in the selection of embryos for transfer improve pregnancy rates? A randomized controlled trial. *Fertil Steril.* 2016;105:275–285.e210.

Kaser DJ, Bormann CL, Missmer SA, Farland LV, Ginsburg ES, Racowsky C. A pilot randomized controlled trial of Day 3 single embryo transfer with adjunctive time-lapse selection versus Day 5 single embryo transfer with or without adjunctive time-lapse selection. *Hum Reprod.* 2017;32:1598–1603.

Kovacic B, Taborin M, Vlaisavljevic V. Artificial blastocoel collapse of human blastocysts before vitrification and its effect on re-expansion after warming – a prospective observational study using time-lapse microscopy. *Reprod Biomed Online.* 2018;36:121–129.

Kovacs P, Lieman HJ. Which embryo selection method should be offered to the patients? *J Assist Reprod Genet.* 2019; 36:603–605.

Li R, Pedersen KS, Liu Y, et al. Effect of red light on the development and quality of mammalian embryos. *J Assist Reprod Genet.* 2014;31:795–801.

Liu Y, Chapple V, Feenan K, Roberts P, Matson P. Time-lapse deselection model for human day 3 in vitro fertilization embryos: the combination of qualitative and quantitative measures of embryo growth. *Fert Ster.* 2016;105:656–662 e651.

Martínez M, Santaló J, Rodríguez A, Vassena R. High reliability of morphokinetic annotations among embryologists. *Hum Reprod Open.* 2018;3: hoy009.

Martinez-Granados L, Serrano M, Gonzalez-Utor A, et al. Inter-laboratory agreement on embryo classification and clinical decision: Conventional morphological assessment vs. time lapse. *PloS One.* 2017;12:e0183328.

Meseguer M, Herrero J, Tejera A, Hilligsoe KM, Ramsing NB, Remohi J. The use of morphokinetics as a predictor of embryo implantation. *Hum Reprod.* 2011;26: 2658–2671.

Petersen BM, Boel M, Montag M, Gardner DK. Development of a generally applicable morphokinetic algorithm capable of predicting the implantation potential of embryos transferred on Day 3. *Hum Reprod.* 2016;31: 2231–2244.

Pribenszky C, Nilselid AM, Montag M. Time-lapse culture with morphokinetic embryo selection improves pregnancy and live birth chances and reduces early pregnancy loss: a meta-analysis. *Reprod Biomed Online.* 2017;35:511–520.

Reignier A, Lammers J, Barriere P, Freour T. Can time-lapse parameters predict embryo ploidy? A systematic review. *Reprod Biomed Online.* 2018;36:380–387.

Rocafort E, Enciso M, Leza A, Sarasa J, Aizpurua J. Euploid embryos selected by an automated time-lapse system have superior SET outcomes than selected solely by conventional morphology assessment. *J Assist Reprod Genet.* 2018;35:1573–1583.

Rubio I, Kuhlmann R, Agerholm I, et al. Limited implantation success of direct-cleaved human zygotes: a time-lapse study. *Fertil Steril.* 2012;98:1458–1463.

Sundvall L, Ingerslev HJ, Breth Knudsen U, Kirkegaard K. Inter- and intra-observer variability of time-lapse annotations. *Human Reprod.* 2013;28:3215–3221.

Tran D, Cooke S, Illingworth PJ, Gardner DK. Deep learning as a predictive tool for fetal heart pregnancy following time-lapse incubation and blastocyst transfer. *Hum Reprod.* 2019;34:1011–1018.

Treff NR, Zimmerman RS. Advances in preimplantation genetic testing for monogenic disease and aneuploidy. *Annu Rev Genomics Hum Genet.* 2017;18:189–200.

VerMilyea MD, Tan L, Anthony JT, et al. Computer-automated time-lapse analysis results correlate with embryo implantation and clinical pregnancy: a blinded, multi-centre study. *Reprod Biomed Online.* 2014;29:729–736

Yang L, Cai S, Zhang S, et al. Single embryo transfer by Day 3 time-lapse selection versus Day 5 conventional morphological selection: a randomized, open-label, non-inferiority trial. *Hum Reprod.* 2018;33:869–876.

Zaninovic N, Irani M, Meseguer M. Assessment of embryo morphology and developmental dynamics by time-lapse microscopy: is there a relation to implantation and ploidy? *Fertil Steril.* 2017;108:722–729.

Zhan Q, Ye Z, Clarke R, Rosenwaks Z, Zaninovic N. Direct unequal cleavages: embryo developmental competence, genetic constitution and clinical outcome. *PLoS One.* 2016;11:e0166398.

Laboratory Monitoring for Embryo Culture

Carlotta Zacà, Andrea Borini, and Giovanni Coticchio

10.1 Introduction

The IVF laboratory is central to Medically Assisted Reproduction perhaps representing also the most crucial extrinsic factor in determining success or failure of treatment. Current science and technology are unable to improve the intrinsic developmental potential of gametes. Therefore, the "mission" of the IVF laboratory consists in the ability to preserve the innate characteristics of sperm and oocytes in the course of preimplantation development and minimize the possible detrimental impact of diverse forms of manipulation. To this end, during culture and manipulation, physical factors (e.g., temperature, atmosphere composition) and stressors (e.g., oocyte microinjection, embryo biopsy) should be monitored and controlled, in order to guarantee stability of conditions considered to be the most appropriate to support and facilitate gamete and embryo function in vitro. In this scenario, the human factor and effectiveness of technical equipment contribute in similar or equivalent proportions in determining clinical outcome. In light of this, not only is monitoring of working conditions of equipment important, but objective assessment of key segments of the IVF process is vital. Performance indicators respond to this need, offering specific, important, and objective measurements of essential processes, such as fertilization, development to blastocyst stage, and cryopreservation. Thus, critical analysis and interpretation of indicators can lead to consistency of results and continued improvement.

10.2 Monitoring

10.2.1 Culture Conditions

In vivo, the microenvironment provides ideal homeostatic conditions for preimplantation development. However, the scenario is completely different when the in vitro-derived embryo develops in a culture droplet placed in a Petri dish. Several physical parameters need to be controlled for carefully to obtain a healthy embryo in vitro. Providing and maintaining proper culture conditions is crucial to minimize stress imposed upon gametes and embryos and to optimize the in-vitro environment.

The major relevant physical parameters are, but not limited to, temperature, pH, osmolarity, humidity, and air quality. (See, e.g., Chapters 2 and 6 for details.)

10.2.1.1 Oxygen

In 1979 an association between mammalian embryo development in vitro and oxygen levels was first reported (Morriss and New, 1979). High and non-physiological oxygen concentrations may have a negative impact through oxidative stress, causing a defective embryo development, with higher rates of fragmentation (Bedaiwy et al., 2004). Conversely, too low oxygen levels may impair embryogenesis, with an involvement of several oxidative processes (Ng et al., 2018). For many years, in human IVF laboratories, atmospheric oxygen tension (~20%) has been used in embryo culture. Therefore, for these reasons, modern IVF incubators should allow monitoring and regulation of oxygen concentration (Swain et al., 2014).

10.2.1.2 Temperature

Temperature is one of the most important factors impacting on IVF outcome. It is well known that temperature can affect gamete and embryo function, particularly meiotic spindle stability (Sun et al., 2004; Wang et al., 2001; Wang et al., 2002) and, under specific conditions, embryo metabolism (Leese et al., 2008).

Laboratory equipment designed to maintain a desired temperature during culture should be subject to daily (if not continuous) monitoring. Indeed, annotation of incubator temperature before start of daily laboratory procedures should be a standard practice. It is common notion that to achieve undisturbed development and desired clinical outcomes, embryos require stable physical conditions when cultured in an incubator (Boone, 2010; Swain, 2014).

During embryo assessment outside the incubator, embryos are exposed to room temperature (Wang, 2002), although great care is normally taken to minimize temperature fluctuations by reducing the time required for observation using warm microscope stages (Magli, 2008).

10.2.1.3 pH and Osmolality

pH is an important regulator of metabolism and other cell functions. Therefore, its dysregulation can severely affect gamete/embryo function and impact IVF outcome. Unlike embryos that have the capacity, although limited, to regulate their internal pH (pHi), oocytes have no robust regulatory mechanisms. Therefore, careful control and monitoring of external pH (pHe) at isolated time points, i.e., testing samples of culture medium exposed to the same conditions, is imperative in IVF (Swain, 2010).

For culture in vitro, pH buffers have been included in the formulation of media to help stabilize pHe (Will et al., 2011) and thereby minimize deleterious intracellular changes arising from fluctuations in pHi (Phillips et al., 2000).

The capacity of embryos to regulate pHi emerges from various studies showing that embryos can be cultured over a pHe range of pH 7.0–7.4 in the absence of significant effects on development (John & Kiessling, 1988; Lane et al., 1998), while deviations of pHe outside this range have shown detrimental effects (Leclerc et al., 1994; Zhao & Baltz, 1996; Zhao et al., 1995; Lane & Bavister, 1999; Lane et al., 1999a,b). At the moment, the optimal pHe value to achieve in the culture milieu is not known, as also shown by the wide range of pHe reported in information sheets of different commercial media.

Another key parameter is osmolality, which should range from 280 to 285 mOsm/kg of water. This information is provided by the manufacturers and considered reliable. However, independent measurement may be required when different solutions are mixed, e.g., when volumes of concentrated protein solutions are diluted in protein-free culture media. Osmolality over 300 mOsm/kg can inhibit embryo development, although this effect may be mitigated by amino acids that act as osmolytes (Swain, 2019).

10.2.1.4 Humidity

Humidity of the incubator environment can be a significant factor in determining IVF outcome. Both for oocyte and embryo culture, 90–100% humidity is considered optimal in an incubator environment.

Appropriate humidity levels minimize the risk of water evaporation from culture drops. If medium evaporation occurs, pH and solute concentrations increase and embryos are no longer exposed to the same solute concentrations initially present in the culture microenvironment. This possible change in osmolality can have detrimental consequences for embryo development (Lane et al., 2008; Swain et al., 2012).

Therefore, the more appropriate and specific conditions to prevent water evaporation from culture drops should be identified and adopted for every laboratory.

10.2.1.5 Air Quality

An additional environmental factor that impacts embryo culture conditions is air quality. Presence and abundance of volatile organic compounds (VOCs) in the laboratory and/or in the incubator may compromise embryo development in terms of cleavage rate and implantation potential (Cohen et al., 1997; Hall et al., 1998; Merton et al., 2007; Khoudja et al., 2013).

VOCs have been detected in gas supply tanks used for IVF incubators (Hall et al., 1998). In such cases, filtering the gases through inline filters before entering the incubator may be an effective approach to improve incubator atmosphere. These filters not only contain HEPA filtration systems to reduce particle counts, but they can also reduce VOC through activated charcoal- or potassium permanganate-based filters.

In this regard, periodic checks of particle count, VOCs, filter integrity, and microbial count should be carried out, in areas where gametes and embryos are handled.

10.3 Performance Indicators

The role of the IVF laboratory in the overall process of MAR is fundamental, involving procurement, preparation, and measurement techniques, aiming at generating a biological product (the embryo) from processing of cells types (the male and female gametes). This procedure in vitro is highly sensitive to extrinsic conditions and also profoundly affected by patient characteristics. For these reasons it has been difficult to standardize and to measure performance in a structured fashion. There have been some efforts by national societies to set standards for benchmarking. For example, the Association of Clinical Embryologists defined several performance indicators for the IVF laboratory, although in a document more generally dedicated to IVF good practice and guidelines (Hughes et al., 2012). In 2012, performance indicators for gamete and embryo cryopreservation were described in a consensus paper published by Alpha Scientists in Reproductive Medicine (2012). In 2017 a consensus document, from ESHRE and Alpha Scientists in Reproductive Medicine, reporting performance indicators (PI) applicable to the mainstream process of the IVF laboratory was published (ESHRE Special Interest Group of Embryology and Alpha Scientists in Reproductive Medicine, 2017). In 2018, ASEBIR (the Spanish embryology association) critically assessed the above cited ESHRE–Alpha document (Lopez-Regalado et al., 2018), stating that some competence levels were not realistic and not based on state-of-the-art performance. In addition, they suggested inclusion of more variables, e.g., embryo utilization rate.

10.3.1 Definition and Characteristics of Performance Indicators

Within the general framework of a Quality Management System (QMS), PIs are measurable parameters to assess the quality of essential healthcare objectives; e.g., patient safety, treatment efficacy, and efficiency. In the specific context of a clinical laboratory, PIs are required to appraise the laboratory's specific contribution to patient treatment.

In order to provide significant information and be generated routinely, any PI should respond to several criteria:

- Coverage of the most important phases of the process occurring in the IVF laboratory
- Definition of specific biological or technical step to be monitored
- Identification of qualifiers (e.g., female age), confounders (e.g., day of embryo transfer), and endpoints (e.g., development to blastocyst stage)
- Reliability and ease of measurement

- Ease of data collection
- Numerical expression by an unambiguous and predetermined formula.

Among PIs, key performance indicators (KPIs) are especially important to:

- Assist in the introduction of a new technique or process
- Define minimum proficiency standards
- Monitor laboratory performance over time
- Define internal quality control and external quality assurance programs
- Set benchmark and quality improvement objectives.

10.3.2 General Recommendations for Indicators of Fresh MAR Treatments

10.3.2.1 Frequency

In clinics with steady and high workload, indicators should be collected monthly. However, in clinics with low monthly activity, such a time interval is not applicable because PI values would not be reliable. Therefore, longer periods between consecutive measurements or a minimum number of treatments (at least 30) should be considered, depending on the stability of the indicator in question.

10.3.2.2 Types of Indicator

Based on their importance and relevance, indicators of the IVF laboratory may be classified into:

i. Reference indicators: relevant to patient response to ovarian stimulation, thereby potentially able to provide indirect information on oocyte quality.

o Proportion of oocytes recovered (stimulated cycles)

o Proportion of MII oocytes at ICSI.

ii. PIs: relatively less important and therefore not necessary to be reported in control charts, but should be documented and stored.

o Sperm motility post-preparation (for IVF and intrauterine insemination)

o IVF polyspermy rate

o 1 PN rate (IVF)

o 1 PN rate (ICSI)

o Good blastocyst development rate.

iii. KPIs: crucial to monitor the most important steps of the IVF process and therefore demanding careful analysis.

- o ICSI damage rate
- o ICSI normal fertilization rate (2PN and 2PB)
- o IVF normal fertilization rate (2PN and 2PB)
- o Failed fertilization rate (IVF)
- o Cleavage rate (day 2)
- o Day 2 Embryo development rate (4-cells)
- o Day 3 Embryo development rate (8-cells)
- o Blastocyst development rate (day 5)
- o Successful biopsy rate
- o Blastocyst cryosurvival rate
- o Implantation rate (cleavage-stage)
- o Implantation rate (blastocyst-stage).

Notably, different KPIs have different significance and reliability. For example; ICSI damage/fertilization rates are very reliable and informative of operator performance; IVF fertilization rates are more relevant to gamete quality and handling; cleavage and blastocyst development rates are very informative of the performance of the culture system; implantation rates, although very important, are less reliable because more influenced by the typology of the reference population, as well as clinical protocols and procedures.

10.3.2.3 Reporting

Indicators should be reported and assessed in relation to proficiency and benchmark values that define a "desirable range" for the laboratory performance.

10.3.2.4 Influence of Clinical and Laboratory Procedures

Clinical (e.g., time of oocyte retrieval from trigger of final maturation, typically 36–38 hours) or laboratory (timing of embryo assessment) procedures can impact the value of indicators. Such factors should be taken into consideration.

10.3.2.5 Reference Population

Several indicators are certainly influenced by the characteristics of the patient population from which they are collected. The ESHRE/Alpha consensus document identified a "reference population" responding to the following criteria:

- female patients <40 years old
- own fresh oocytes
- ejaculated spermatozoa (fresh or frozen)

- no PGT
- both insemination methods (i.e. standard IVF and ICSI).

Individual clinics may opt for a different (or multiple) reference population that may better represent the typology of their patient.

10.3.3 Indicators of Cryopreserved MAR Treatments

KPIs for cryopreserved MAR treatments were published by Alpha Scientists in Reproductive Medicine in 2012 (Alpha Scientists in Reproductive Medicine, 2012). Most of the general criteria of definition, characteristics, and recommendations reported above and relevant to fresh treatments are also applicable to cryopreservation PIs. Such indicators are divided into categories relevant to the use of cryopreserved oocytes, zygotes, cleavage-stage, and blastocyst-stage embryos.

a. Oocyte KPIs

    i. Morphological survival
    ii. Fertilization rate
    iii. Embryo development rate
    iv. Implantation rate

b. Zygote KPIs

    i. Morphological survival
    ii. Cleavage rate
    iii. Embryo development rate
    iv. Implantation rate

c. Embryo KPIs

    i. Morphological survival: fully intact
    ii. Morphological survival: ≥50% intact
    iii. Post-warming embryo development rate (if applicable)
    iv. Implantation rate

d. Blastocyst KPIs

    i. Morphological survival
    ii. Embryo transfer rate
    iii. Implantation rate

Like PIs of fresh treatments, cryopreservation PIs relevant to survival and subsequent development of oocytes and embryos should be reported and appraised in comparison with "desirable ranges" of laboratory performance defined by proficiency and benchmark values. Importantly, such proficiency and benchmark values are different depending or whether gametes/embryos are cryopreserved by slow freezing or vitrification. However, cryopreservation KPIs are based on evidence or empirical experience generated until 2010, i.e., a period when vitrification had been already introduced on quite a large scale, but not probably optimized. Since then, vitrification has experienced further expansion and standardization. In the light of such progress, some proficiency or benchmark values appear inappropriate in consideration of current standards of performance. For example, in the Alpha consensus document, the competence (proficiency) value of blastocyst survival rate after cryopreservation by vitrification is 80%, clearly inadequate to appraise the current standard of performance of blastocyst cryopreservation in the large majority of laboratories worldwide. Similarly, a survival rate of 70% as competence value for oocyte vitrification appears too low compared with data reported in publications of the last several years. More generally, assessment of oocyte survival rate may be particularly prone to error. For example, for a given cohort of oocytes this rate may vary significantly depending on whether morphological viability is assessed shortly after the warming procedure or 60–90 minutes later. Therefore, while the Alpha cryopreservation KPIs document has been instrumental in measuring laboratory performance and, more generally, in introducing a methodology for objective evaluation, significant progress in oocyte and embryo cryopreservation calls for a review of proficiency and benchmark values.

10.4 Troubleshooting

Measurement and regular monitoring of KPIs is extremely important to identify and manage factors that may have a negative or (less frequently) positive impact on the overall IVF laboratory performance. There are countless possible situations. A decrease in implantation rate could be caused by a myriad of intrinsic (e.g., a change in patient population despite its definition a priori) or extrinsic (e.g., materials, protocol application) factors. For example, several years ago, in some IVF laboratories in Europe, a significant decrease in day 2 embryo cleavage rate was detected (by authors). By prompt identification of an embryotoxic effect associated with an albumin batch used for culture media production, an early

warning addressed to laboratories and manufacturers prevented further use of this culture medium, reducing a wider impact on clinical outcome. Other possible examples of troubleshooting may concern any step of the IVF process. An increase in the rate of 3PN may indicate a shift in the timing of ICSI in relation to the stage of oocyte maturation; i.e., if ICSI is performed too early, oocytes classified as metaphase II because displaying the second polar body may be in fact still engaged in telophase II, with the consequence that maternal sister chromatids are retained in the oocyte and a third polar body is formed. Alternatively, if an increase in 2PN rate associated with a specific ICSI operator is consistently detected, then the technical factor responsible for such increase should be identified and systematically adopted by all operators. In a recent publication by Hammond and Morbeck (2019), a negative impact after a switch of culture media could be identified by use of a statistical KPI monitoring system.

10.5 Future Evolution of (K)PIs

Current KPIs are very valuable assessment tools that should be adopted systematically to track performance and quality of IVF laboratories. However, novel PIs may be developed. For example, time lapse technology provides a unique opportunity to increase the sensitivity of PIs relevant to embryo development. In this respect, it has been shown that by adopting morphokinetic algorithms it is possible to detect culture media toxicants that otherwise would go unnoticed using a standard mouse embryo assay based on simple blastocyst development rate (Wolff et al., 2013). Novel KPIs may also be required following an increase in the use of a given procedure. In the field of cryopreservation, blastocyst vitrification has become increasingly popular over the last 15 years. Because at this stage single cells cannot be discriminated and therefore the degree of possible postwarming embryo damage cannot be precisely determined, a possible proxy for embryo viability could be represented by blastocyst re-expansion within a given time interval (Ahlström et al., 2013). Further potential of using morphokinetics for KPIs has not yet been explored.

10.6 Summary

- Until a decade ago, the need to measure IVF laboratory performance indicators was recognized but measurements were not being performed in a structured manner.

- PIs are measurable parameters to assess the quality of essential healthcare objectives and therefore applicable to the IVF process.

- Among PIs, key performance indicators (KPIs) are especially important to: assist in the introduction of a new technique or process; define minimum proficiency standards; monitor laboratory performance; define internal quality control and external quality assurance programs.

- During the past decade, national and international societies have elaborated PIs for the IVF process and cryopreservation.

- Essential elements for the definition of PIs in IVF are: frequency of measurement; type of KI, reporting; control of laboratory and clinical variables; reference population.

- A separate set of PIs is dedicated to cryopreserved oocytes and embryos.

- KIs should be implemented not only to the aim of assuring consistency of the IVF laboratory performance, but also to identify factors with a positive or a negative impact on outcome that have been introduced unintentionally in the process.

- Novel PIs should be constantly searched for, exploiting newly introduced technologies.

References

Alpha Scientists in Reproductive Medicine. The Alpha consensus meeting on cryopreservation key performance indicators and benchmarks: proceedings of an expert meeting. *Reprod Biomed Online.* 2012;25: 146–167.

Ahlström A, Westin C, Wikland M, Hardarson T. Prediction of live birth in frozen-thawed single blastocyst transfer cycles by pre-freeze and post-thaw morphology. *Hum Reprod.* 2013;28:1199–1209.

Armstrong S, Arroll N, Cree LM, Jordan V, Farquhar C. Time-lapse systems for embryo incubation and assessment in assisted reproduction. *Cochrane Database Syst Rev.* 2015;5(5):CD011320.

Bavister B. Oxygen concentration and preimplantation development. *Reprod Biomed Online.* 2004;9: 484–486.

Bedaiwy MA, Falcone T, Mohamed MS, et al. Differential growth of human embryos in vitro: role of reactive oxygen species. *Fertil Steril.* 2004;82:593–600.

Boone WR, Johnson JE, Locke AJ, Crane 4th MM, Price TM. Control of air quality in an assisted reproductive technology laboratory. *Fertil. Steril.* 1999;71:150–154.

Boone WR, Lee Higdon III H, Johson JE. Quality management issues in the assisted reproduction laboratory. *J Reprod Stem Cell Biotechnol.* 2010;1:30–107.

Bontekoe S, Mantikou E, van Wely M, Seshadri S, Repping S, Mastenbroek S. Low oxygen concentrations for embryo culture in assisted reproductive technologies. *Cochrane Database Syst. Rev.* 2012;11;7:CD008950.

Cohen J, Gilligan A, Esposito W, Schimmel T, Dale B. Ambient air and its potential effects on conception in vitro. *Hum Reprod.* 1997;12:1742–1749.

ESHRE Special Interest Group of Embryology, Alpha Scientists In Reproductive Medicine. The Vienna consensus: report of an expert meeting on the development of art laboratory performance indicators. *Hum Reprod Open.* 2017;35:494–510.

Esteves SC, Verza Jr, S, Gomes AP. Comparison between international standard organization (ISO) type 5 and type 6 cleanrooms combined with volatile organic compounds filtration system for micromanipulation and embryo culture in severe male factor infertility. *Fertil Steril.* 2006;86: S353–S354.

Fawzy M, AbdelRahman MY, Zidan MH, et al. Humid versus dry incubator: a prospective, randomized, controlled trial. *Fertil Steril.* 2017;108:277–283.

Fischer B, Bavister BD. Oxygen tension in the oviduct and uterus of rhesus monkeys, hamsters and rabbits. *J Reprod Fertil.* 1993;99:673–679.

Goto Y, Noda Y, Mori T, Nakano M. Increased generation of reactive oxygen species in embryos cultured in vitro. *Free Radic Biol Med.* 1993;15:69–75.

Hall J, Gilligan A, Schimmel T, Cecchi M, Cohen J. The origin, effects and control of air pollution in laboratories used for human embryo culture. *Hum Reprod.* 1998;13:146–155.

Hammond ER, Morbeck DE. Tracking quality: can embryology key performance indicators be used to identify clinically relevant shifts in pregnancy rate? *Hum Reprod.,* 2019;34:37–43.

Higdon 3rd HL, Blackhurst DW, Boone WR. Incubator management in an assisted reproductive technology laboratory. *Fertil Steril.* 2008;89:703–710.

Hong K, Forman E, Lee H, Ferry K, Treff N, Scott R. Optimizing the temperature for embryo culture in

IVF: a randomized controlled trial (RCT) comparing standard culture temperature of 37°C to the reduced more physiologic temperature of 36°C. *Fertil Steril.* 2012;98, s167.

Hughes C, Association of Clinical Embryologists. Association of clinical embryologists – guidelines on good practice in clinical embryology laboratories 2012. *Hum Fertil.* 2012;15:174–189.

Hunter RH. Temperature gradients in female reproductive tissues. *Reprod Biomed Online.* 2012;24:377–380.

Hunter RH, Einer-Jensen N. Pre-ovulatory temperature gradients within mammalian ovaries: a review. *J Anim Physiol Anim Nutr. (Berl.)* 2005;89:240–243.

Hunter RH, Einer-Jensen N, Greve T. Presence and significance of temperature gradients among different ovarian tissues. *Microsc Res Tech.* 2006;69:501–507.

Iwata K, Yumoto K, Mio Y. Unstable osmotic pressure in microdrops cultured under mineral oil in non-humidified incubators. *Fertil Steril.* 2016;106:e355.

John DP, Kiessling AA. Improved pronuclear mouse embryo development over an extended pH range in Ham's F-10 medium without protein. *Fertil Steril.* 1988;49:150–155.

Khoudja RY, Xu Y, Li T, Zhou C. Better IVF outcomes following improvements in laboratory air quality. *J Assist Reprod Genet.* 2013;30:69–76.

Kovacic B, Vlaisavljevic V. Influence of atmospheric versus reduced oxygen concentration on development of human blastocysts in vitro: a prospective study on sibling oocytes. *Reprod Biomed Online.* 2008;17:229–236.

Lane M, Baltz JM, Bavister BD. Regulation of intracellular pH in hamster preimplantation embryos by the sodium hydrogen (Na+/ H

+) antiporter. *Biol Reprod.* 1998;59:1483–1490.

Bicarbonate/chloride exchange regulates intracellular pH of embryos but not oocytes of the hamster. *Biol Reprod.* 1999a;61:452–457.

Na+/H+ antiporter activity in hamster embryos is activated during fertilization. *Dev Biol.* 1999b;208:244–252.

Lane M, Bavister BD. Regulation of intracellular pH in bovine oocytes and cleavage stage embryos. *Mol Reprod Dev.* 1999;54:396–401.

Lane M, Mitchell M, Cashman KS, Feil D, Wakefield S, Zander-Fox DL. To QC or not to QC: The key to a consistent laboratory. *Reprod Fertil Dev.* 2008;20:23–32.

Leclerc C, Becker D, Buehr M, Warner A. Low intracellular pH is involved in the early embryonic death of DDK mouse eggs fertilized by alien sperm. *Dev Dyn.* 1994;200:257–267.

Leese HJ, Baumann CG, Brison DR, McEvoy TG, Sturmey RG. Metabolism of the viable mammalian embryo: quietness revisited. *Mol Hum Reprod.* 2008;14:667–672.

Li R, Pedersen KS, Liu Y, et al. Effect of red light on the development and quality of mammalian embryos. *J Assist Reprod Genet.* 2014;31:795–801.

Lopez-Regalado ML, Martínez-Granados L, González-Utor A, et al. Critical appraisal of the Vienna consensus: performance indicators for assisted reproductive technology laboratories. *Reprod Biomed Online.* 2018;37:128–132.

Magli MC, Van den Abbeel E, Lundin K, et al. Revised guidelines for good practice in IVF laboratories. *Hum Reprod.* 2008;23:1253–1262.

Mantikou E, Bontekoe S, van Wely M, Seshadri S, Repping S, Mastenbroek S. Low oxygen concentrations for embryo culture

in assisted reproductive technologies. *Hum Reprod Update.* 2013;19:209.

McKiernan SH, Bavister BD. Environmental variables influencing in vitro development of hamster 2-cell embryos to the blastocyst stage. *Biol Reprod.* 1990;43:404–413.

Meintjes M, Chantilis SJ, Douglas JD, et al. A controlled randomized trial evaluating the effect of lowered incubator oxygen tension on live births in a predominantly blastocyst transfer program. *Hum Reprod.* 2009;24:300–307.

Merton JS, Vermeulen ZL, Otter T, Mullaart E, de Ruigh L, Hasler JF. Carbon-activated gas filtration during in vitro culture increased pregnancy rate following transfer of in vitro-produced bovine embryos. *Theriogenology* 2007;67:1233–1238.

Meseguer M, Rubio I, Cruz M, Basile N, Marcos J, Requena A. Embryo incubation and selection in a time-lapse monitoring system improves pregnancy outcome compared with a standard incubator: a retrospective cohort study. *Fertil Steril.* 2012;98:1481–1489.e1410.

Morbeck DE. Air quality in the assisted reproduction laboratory: a mini-review. *J Assist Reprod Genet.* 2015;32:1019–1024.

Morriss GM, New DA. Effect of oxygen concentration on morphogenesis of cranial neural folds and neural crest in cultured rat embryos. *J Embryol Exp Morphol.* 1979;54:17–35.

Nakahara T, Iwase A, Goto M, Harata T, Suzuki M, Ienaga M, et al. Evaluation of the safety of time-lapse observations for human embryos. *J Assist Reprod Genet.* 2010;27:93–96.

Ng KYB, Mingels R, Morgan H, Macklon N, Cheong Y. In vivo oxygen, temperature and pH dynamics in the female reproductive tract and their importance in human conception: a systematic review. *Hum Reprod Update.* 2018;24:15–34.

Olds S, Stemm K, Wachter K, Wiemer K. Analysis of embryo culture media pH changes during incubator use and media evaporation under oil using a continous pH monitoring system. *Fertil Steril.* 2015;104:e318–e319.

Pabon JE Jr, Findley WE, Gibbons WE. The toxic effect of short exposures to the atmospheric oxygen concentration on early mouse embryonic development. *Fertil Steril.* 1989;51:896–900.

Phillips KP, Leveille MC, Claman P, Baltz JM. Intracellular pH regulation in human preimplantation embryos. *Hum Reprod.* 2000;15:896–904.

Quinn P, Harlow GM. The effect of oxygen on the development of preimplantation mouse embryos in vitro. *J Exp Zool.* 1978;206:73–80.

Sun XF, Wang WH, Keefe DL. Overheating is detrimental to meiotic spindles within in vitro matured human oocytes. *Zygote.* 2004;12:65–70.

Swain JE. Optimizing the culture environment in the IVF laboratory: impact of pH and buffer capacity on gamete and embryo quality. *Reprod Biomed Online.* 2010;21:6–16.

Decisions for the IVF laboratory: comparative analysis of embryo culture incubators. *Reprod Biomed Online* 2014;28:535–547.

Optimal human embryo culture. *Semin Reprod Med* 2015;33:103–117.

Controversies in ART: considerations and risks for uninterrupted embryo culture. *Reprod Biomed Online.* 2019;39:19–26.

Swain JE, Cabrera L, Xu X, Smith GD. Microdrop preparation factors influence culture-media osmolality, which can impair mouse embryo preimplantation development. *Reprod Biomed Online.* 2012;24:142–147.

Swain J, Graham C, Kile R, Schoolcraft WB, Krisher R. Media evaporation in a dry culture incubator; effect of dish, drop size and oil on media osmolality. *Fertil Steril.* 2018;110:e363–e364.

Umaoka Y, Noda Y, Narimoto K, Mori T. Effects of oxygen toxicity on early development of mouse embryos. *Mol Reprod Dev.* 1992;31:28–33.

Waldenstrom U, Engstrom AB, Hellberg D, Nilsson S. Low-oxygen compared with high-oxygen atmosphere in blastocyst culture, a prospective randomized study. *Fertil Steril.* 2009;91:2461–2465.

Wang WH, Meng L, Hackett RJ, Odenbourg R, Keefe DL. Limited recovery of meiotic spindles in living human oocytes after cooling-rewarming observed using polarized light microscopy. *Hum Reprod.* 2001;16:2374–2378.

Wang WH, Meng L, Hackett RJ, Oldenbourg R, Keefe DL. Rigorous thermal control during intracytoplasmic sperm injection stabilizes the meiotic spindle and improves fertilization and pregnancy rates. *Fertil Steril.* 2002;77:1274–1277.

Will MA, Clark NA, Swain JE. Biological pH buffers in IVF: help or hindrance to success. *J Assist Reprod Genet.* 2011;28:711–724.

Wolff HS, Fredrickson JR, Walker DL, Morbeck DE. Advances in quality control: mouse embryo morphokinetics are sensitive markers of in vitro stress. *Hum Reprod.* 2013;28:1776–1782.

Zhang JQ, Li XL, Peng Y, Guo X, Heng BC, Tong GQ. Reduction in exposure of human embryos outside the incubator enhances embryo quality and blastulation rate. *Reprod Biomed Online.* 2010;20:510–515.

Zhao Y, Baltz JM. Bicarbonate/chloride exchange and intracellular pH throughout preimplantation mouse embryo development. *Am J Physiol.* 1996;271:C1512–C1520.

Zhao Y, Chauvet PJ, Alper SL, Baltz JM. Expression and function of bicarbonate/chloride exchangers in the preimplantation mouse embryo. *J Biol Chem.* 1995;270:24428–24434.

Embryo Culture and IVF Offspring Outcome

John Dumoulin and Aafke van Montfoort

11.1 Introduction

Since the birth of Louise Brown, the first 'test tube baby', in 1978, assisted reproductive technology (ART) has become one of the standard treatments for couples with subfertility problems. Today, it is estimated that 8 million children have been born via ART worldwide and up to 6% of newborns in Europe are conceived via this technique (Adamson et al., 2019). Surprisingly, relatively little is known about the short- and especially long-term effects of ART manipulations on the health risks for the children.

In the beginning of IVF, multiple embryos were transferred to increase the chance of live birth. This practice resulted in a high rate of multiple pregnancies, with the inherent increased risk for preterm birth, low birthweight, and other health problems. The transition towards single embryo transfer (SET) decreased the multiple birth rate considerably and concomitantly the perinatal risks for ART children decreased as well. Nevertheless, a smaller, but still increased risk remained in singleton ART children. Berntsen et al. (2019) summarized the outcomes of the large cohort studies and meta-analyses. The results of the studies are consistent, showing an increased risk for preterm birth (adjusted risk (AR) 1.41–2.04), very preterm birth (AR 1.68–3.07), low birthweight (AR 1.6–1.7), very low birthweight (AR 1.8–3.0), small for gestational age (AR around 1.5), and perinatal mortality (AR 1.7–2.0) when compared to spontaneous conceptions. Alongside, an increased risk for obstetric complications, such as gestational diabetes, pregnancy related hypertension, placenta praevia, and abruption and preterm rupture of membranes is reported (Berntsen et al., 2019). The adverse perinatal outcomes are to a large part attributable to subfertility-related factors in the parents, as the risk for these outcomes is higher in spontaneously conceived women with a time to pregnancy of more than 1 year as compared to less than 1 year (Pinborg et al., 2013). However, among siblings, the child conceived via ART has a poorer perinatal outcome than the child conceived spontaneously. This implies that ART related manipulations also play an important role.

Studies investigating long-term health effects are largely reassuring as no increase or no consistently reported increase in malignancies, adverse neurodevelopmental health outcomes, or growth alterations have been reported (Berntsen et al., 2019). However, the cardiovascular health of ART offspring deserves attention. In a meta-analysis, including 872 IVF-ICSI offspring and 3034 spontaneously conceived offspring, the systolic and diastolic blood pressure of ART offspring was 1.88 (95% CI 0.27–3.49) and 1.51 (95% CI 0.33–2.70) mmHg higher, respectively. When stratifying the analysis according to decade in which the children were born, the higher blood pressure was only present in the older cohorts born between 1990 and 1999 and not in the more recent cohorts born between 2000 and 2009 (Guo et al., 2017). On the other hand, in five studies in which a large proportion of children were born in the 20th century, suboptimal cardiac diastolic function and cardiovascular morphology, such as intima media, thickness were reported (Guo et al., 2017). As ART offspring are growing older, future will reveal if these cardiovascular findings are evident in ART-conceived adults.

These reported adverse perinatal outcomes together with the cardiovascular alterations are reasons for concern as it is known from other non-IVF related cohorts, starting with the landmark studies from Professors Barker and Osmond, that prematurity and low birthweight are associated with an increased risk for long-term health effects, such as cardiovascular diseases (Roseboom, 2018). This association is captured in the developmental origins of health and disease (DOHaD) hypothesis. Low birthweight is seen as an indicator of altered fetal growth and other adaptations (programming) that might affect long-term health and disease. Environmental exposures during pregnancy, but possibly also during early embryonic development, may lead to adaptations in the physiology and metabolism of organs and cells. These adaptations are in all probability beneficial for the short term, but may increase the vulnerability for diseases in later life. An illustrative example comes from people exposed in utero to the Dutch famine in World War II. When exposed early in pregnancy, they had a similar birthweight as non-exposed, but a doubled risk for cardiovascular disease in later life (Roseboom, 2018). In animals, nutritional changes during the few days around conception only, already lead to long-term health effects in the offspring, such as impaired glucose tolerance and cardiovascular dysfunction (Roseboom, 2018). Altogether, this makes it plausible that IVF children could be at risk and urges for research into the health effects of IVF on the children, the specific parts of IVF that are causative, and the mechanisms by which these programming processes work.

Obtaining reliable results from human follow-up studies is, however, not so obvious, given the (methodological) issues associated with these kind of studies. These include the retrospective design of most studies and the small sample sizes (while large numbers are needed to detect the relative small differences that are to be expected). Furthermore, phenotypic and/or health parameters such as birthweight, child growth, cognitive development, and cardiometabolic parameters are subject to many confounding factors, such as socioeconomic status and lifestyle, as well as genetic factors for which correction is not always possible. Inherently associated with human ART follow-up studies are the absence of 'old' ART cohorts as the technique is relatively young and the parental subfertility that always interferes when studying effects of ART procedures. Finally, a risk for publication bias exists as studies that do find an association between ART and health outcome parameters will be published more readily.

Given these challenges, animal studies can prove to be valuable with respect to unraveling potential health effects of ART-related procedures. One of the most important advantages is that patient-related confounding factors, such as subfertility, genetics, and lifestyle (Pinborg et al., 2013), are of no importance in animal studies. However, it must be realized that differences between species and in ART protocols make it difficult to deduce definitive answers. For example, in domestic animals (cattle, sheep, horses) embryos are obtained from in vitro matured oocytes

while most human ART oocytes mature in vivo. Furthermore, embryos in animal studies are mainly transferred to young fertile recipients in a cycle without superovulation (Duranthon & Chavatte-Palmer, 2018). Also, relatively few studies have been published, concerning the long-term effects of ART procedures on the offspring in animal models, which is perhaps surprising as the shorter lifespan would simplify these studies. The limited success and use of ART, resulting in relatively low number of ART offspring produced in many animal models, are likely to be the main causes. We will therefore focus on two animal species in which these problems are least prominent, cattle and mice, to discuss the effects of embryo culture on health of the offspring, and relate to the limited data available from human studies. In the end, we will briefly touch upon possible programming mechanisms that are affected by embryo culture.

11.2 Embryo Culture and IVF Offspring Outcome – Animal Studies

In cattle, ART is widely used to accelerate the genetic improvement in breeding programs and almost a million embryos are produced yearly (Duranthon & Chavatte-Palmer, 2018; Ealy et al., 2019). The independent effect of in vitro culture is difficult to derive as most studies in cattle use in vitro produced (IVP) embryos that usually originate from in vitro matured oocytes that are fertilized and cultured in vitro to the blastocyst stage (Duranthon & Chavatte-Palmer, 2018). In vitro production affects the success rates in terms of live born calves after transfer (Wondim et al., 2014; Duranthon & Chavatte-Palmer, 2018; Salilew-Vrooman & Bartolomei, 2017, Wrenzycki, 2018; Ealy et al., 2019). Pregnancy rates are 10–40% lower compared to superovulation only and pregnancy losses are higher, ranging from 60% to 85%, compared to 10–65% for in vivo produced embryos after artificial insemination.

Morphokinetic differences exist between IVP and in vivo-generated conceptuses during the peri-attachment period (day 12–20 of gestation), as well as differences in molecules secreted by the conceptus and the maternal endometrium during their interaction at implantation. In early gestation, IVP fetuses are reduced in size compared to fetuses after in vivo conception, while in late gestation, IVP fetuses are generally larger. Adverse perinatal outcomes after

IVP, commonly known as the large offspring syndrome, have been reported with birthweights of up to twice the expected weight and a high incidence of congenital abnormalities, such as limb deformities, an enlarged tongue (macroglossia), and heart abnormalities. Neonatal health is also compromised after IVP with increases in the incidences of stillbirth and neonatal death (Duranthon & Chavatte-Palmer, 2018; Ealy et al., 2019).

Few studies describe long-term health effects of IVP up to the adult age, as animals are often sold to clients and/or are culled at a relatively young age. In two studies, IVP-generated calves surviving the neonatal period had normal mortality rates and economic outcome parameters, such as reproductive function and milk production. In another study in which X-sorted semen was used, an increased risk of mortality and reduced milk yield in a subgroup of IVP-generated calves was reported (summarized in Duranthon & Chavatte-Palmer, 2018; Ealy et al., 2019).

Although the reported effects of IVP may be attributed to ART aspects other than the in vitro culture of embryos, suboptimal conditions such as the use of coculture with feeder cells or the presence of serum in culture medium, have shown to induce abnormal perinatal large offspring syndrome phenotype (Ealy et al., 2019).

Rodents such as the rat, rabbit, and especially the mouse have been widely used as models for the evaluation of the effects of ART on fetal development and long-term health of the offspring. Many studies have shown that fetal growth and birthweight are affected when embryos are cultured in vitro during the preimplantation embryo stages, as compared to in vivo developed controls (see Zandstra et al., 2015 for overview). Studies found that in vitro culture could affect postnatal growth and organ size, as well as adult health including glucose metabolism, obesity, cardiovascular health, and behavior, often in a sex- and strain-specific manner (see extensive reviews: Calle et al., 2012; Duranthon & Chavatte-Palmer, 2018; Feuer & Rinaudo, 2017; Gardner & Kelley, 2017; Vrooman & Bartolomei, 2017). However, whether or not these adverse health effects also result in a shortened life span remains to be determined. In one study, no effect of embryo culture was found on longevity of offspring in mice, while in another study, a significantly shorter lifespan was found, but only in combination with being fed a high fat western diet (Feuer & Rinaudo, 2017).

It remains to be determined which of the different ART culture aspects contributes the most to these health effects. It must be realized that during in vitro culture, embryos are exposed to many stressors that are absent or different in the in vivo environment in which they normally develop, such as fluctuations in temperature, oxygen, pH, light exposure, the absence of growth factors and cytokines, the type of protein source used, and the relatively large volume of surrounding medium. However, it is clear that the environment in which embryos are cultured during their preimplantation development can have a profound effect on perinatal and postnatal health. Two aspects of the in vitro environment of embryos are most widely studied: culture media and the oxygen concentration in the gas phase.

Several investigators have studied the effect of specific culture media components on long-term health outcomes. The group of Gutiérrez-Adán studied the effect of supplementing the culture medium with either fetal calf serum (FCS) or bovine serum albumin in a mouse model and found that offspring of the FCS group had a significantly higher body weight and increased liver and heart weight at 20 weeks of age, with females being more affected than males (discussed in Duranthon & Chavatte-Palmer, 2018). The group of Banrezes and Ozil studied the effect of transiently (only 15 hours during the zygote stage) modifying the redox potential by providing only a single exogenous carbohydrate (either pyruvate or lactate) to mouse embryos, which resulted in induced NAD(P)H oxidation and a low mitochondrial activity in the embryos. Significant differences up to the age of 20 weeks were found in the growth profiles of the offspring from the different experimental groups (Duranthon & Chavatte-Palmer, 2018). The group of Fleming studied the effect of supplementing the culture medium with a low concentration of insulin and so-called branched-chain amino acids (BCAA) valine, isoleucine, and leucine. The concentration of insulin and BCAA was chosen to mimic the effect on the insulin level in serum and BCAA level in uterine luminal fluid found in their in vivo model in which females were fed a low protein diet. They found a significant increase in birthweight and weight gain during early postnatal life up to 10 weeks of age. Furthermore, relative hypertension in male offspring was found as well as reduced heart/body weight in female offspring (Velazquez et al., 2018). In addition, accumulated waste products in the culture medium, such as ammonium, have been found to correlate to incidences of neural tube birth defects (Gardner & Kelley, 2017).

The oxygen concentration in the gas phase used during in vitro culture is a second important factor that affects embryo development and perinatal outcome. The concentration of oxygen in the reproductive tract of all investigated species is typically between 2% and 8%, compared to atmospheric oxygen concentration of approximately 20%. Culture of embryos under atmospheric oxygen concentrations has been common practice in the past (and still is in many laboratories today) in both animal and human IVF. As summarized in several studies (Salilew-Wondim et al., 2014; Wale & Gardner, 2016; Gardner & Kelley, 2017; Mani & Mainigi, 2018), culture of preimplantation embryos under the more physiological concentration of 5% oxygen resulted in more optimal development with higher blastocyst rates, higher mean number of cells per blastocyst, and higher fetal development rates in many species including sheep, cow, goat, pig, and mice, as well as humans.

Despite evidence, indications that atmospheric oxygen levels lead to long-term effects are scarce. However, it makes an embryo more susceptible to a second stressor such as suboptimal culture medium, single embryo culture, and/or exposure to ammonium (Feuer & Rinaudo, 2017, Gardner & Kelley, 2017). This was demonstrated in the studies by Feuer and Rinaudo (2017). They cultured mouse embryos in different culture media and oxygen concentrations and found that offspring from embryos that were cultured in Whitten's medium under 20% oxygen had higher body weights and exhibited glucose intolerance at 19 weeks of age compared with control mice (in vivo-derived blastocysts transferred to foster mothers) while offspring from embryos that were cultured in KSOM medium with amino acids under 5% oxygen had a normal postnatal growth and glucose homeostasis (Feuer & Rinaudo, 2017).

11.3 Embryo Culture and IVF Offspring Outcome – Human Studies

11.3.1 Culture Medium

Even though the effects of culture medium on off-spring health were already widely established in animals, it was not until 2010 that the first study showing the effects of culture media on birthweight

in humans was published by our group (Dumoulin et al., 2010). In our IVF center, for quality control purposes, at least two culture media are routinely used in parallel. Between July 2003 and December 2006, Vitrolife G1™ Version 3 (Göteborg, Sweden) and K-SICM from Cook (Brisbane, Australia) were used. Cycles were assigned to one of the two media by strictly alternating consecutive IVF treatments between the two types. Initially, only data from first IVF treatments with fresh embryo transfer were included in the study (see Figure 11.1): 414 cycles in which embryos were cultured in Vitrolife medium and 412 cycles with culture in Cook medium resulted in 110 and 78 live born singletons, respectively. Mean birthweight (in g ± standard error of the mean (SEM)) and birthweight corrected for gestational age and gender (z-score ± SEM) were significantly higher in the Vitrolife group (3453 (± 53) and 0.13 (± 0.09) vs. 3208 (± 61) and -0.31 (± 0.10)). Even after correction for potential confounders, such as height and weight of the parents, parity, pregnancy complications, and maternal smoking, the difference remained significant, although it must be acknowledged that a larger number of live births are needed to confirm these results.

In a later analysis including all fresh embryo transfers that resulted in a singleton live birth in the study period (July 2003 to December 2006) ($n = 168$ in the Vitrolife group and $n = 126$ in the Cook group, Figure 11.1), the birthweight difference was confirmed with a significant adjusted difference of 112 g. Moreover, in the Cook group, the rate of neonates with a low birthweight (<2500 g) was significantly higher. Gestational age was not related to the culture medium used. A retrospective examination of the fetal growth parameters of the 294 singletons, collected during regular pregnancy check-ups, revealed that fetal growth diverges from the second trimester onwards.

Following this first publication, several other comparison studies studying the effects of culture medium have been published. In a review, out of ten studies excluding ours, three showed a significant difference in birthweight (Zandstra et al., 2015). One of these three investigated the effect of the protein source added to the medium on birthweight and the other two each compared different brands of culture media.

Comparison of studies is complicated for several reasons. In the 11 studies in the review, 22 media comparisons were done, with 19 different media

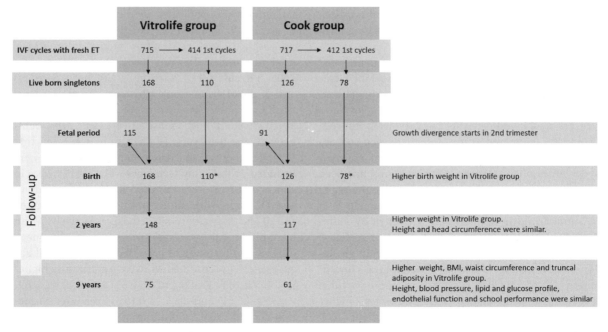

Figure 11.1 Flow chart and outcomes of a cohort of IVF cycles performed between July 2003 and December 2006, when the use of two types of culture media (Vitrolife and Cook) was strictly alternated between consecutive IVF cycles. Only a women's first live born singleton resulting from fresh embryo transfer was included for follow-up. The first paper for this cohort (Dumoulin et al., 2010) described birthweight differences in singletons born from women's first cycles (*). Later, the cohort was expanded with all singletons born. Retrospectively, fetal growth data from these singletons were collected. At 2 and 9 years, this cohort was approached for further follow-up. The numbers indicate the number of included subjects at each stage of follow-up. For color version of this figure. Please refer color plate section.

comparisons. Although it may be assumed that growth effects are related to specific formulations of culture media, the different compositions of the culture media and the lack of manufacturers' information on the exact amount of each component complicates the comparison of the different studies. Furthermore, most studies had a retrospective design comparing two separate time windows in which another medium was used. The influence of other factors that have changed over time, such as population characteristics, stimulation protocols, or other procedures, cannot be excluded. The retrospective design also limited the possibility to properly correct for potential confounders in many studies. To compare neonatal outcomes of two culture media, a substantial number of cycles are needed. For instance, to detect a birthweight difference of 100 g, with a standard deviation of 500 g, $\alpha < 0.05$ and a power of 80%, 393 children in each group are needed. With a hypothesized live birth rate of 25%, 1600 IVF cycles resulting in 400 children are required in each group to prove a 100 g difference in birthweight. This is not always feasible, especially for small IVF centers and because manufacturers might

come up with a new version before the required number of inclusions is completed. To obtain such numbers, multicenter trials are almost a prerequisite.

Recently, in the Netherlands, a multicenter trial was conducted in six IVF centers, where 836 couples were randomized to the use of Vitrolife G5™ or HTF (Lonza) for embryo culture in one fresh cycle and all resulting frozen-embryo transfer cycles performed within 1 year. The primary outcome was cumulative live birth rate (relative risk (RR) Vitrolife vs. HTF = 1.2, 95% CI 0.99–1.37) with birthweight as a secondary outcome. In the 300 live born singleton children in this trial, birthweight was significantly lower in the G5 group compared with the HTF group. The adjusted mean birthweight, adjustment is important here because of the increased prematurity rate in the G5 group, was 116 g lower in the G5 group than in the HTF group (95% CI −212 to −20). Likewise, after exclusion of the preterm births, birthweight remained significantly different. The birthweight divergence must have occurred after 20 weeks of gestation, as the estimated fetal weight at 20 weeks of gestation was similar in both groups (Kleijkers et al., 2016).

To analyze the long term effects of culture medium, we performed follow-up studies of the Vitrolife-Cook cohort at the age of 2 and 9 years. At 2 years of age (Figure 11.1), height, weight, and head circumference data collected at 11 time-points during the first two years of life as part of the children's health program at municipal infant welfare centres in the Netherlands were retrieved. Height and head circumference were similar at all time-points between the two groups. Weight, however, remained higher in the Vitrolife group at all 11 time-points, with most differences being significant. At the age of 2 years, the adjusted difference in weight standard deviation score (SDS) normalized for age and gender was 0.39. The Vitrolife group, with a mean weight SDS score of 0.07 was more comparable to the Dutch reference population than the Cook group with a weight SDS of -0.43 (summarized in Berntsen et al., 2019).

In a further follow-up study at 9 years of age (Figure 11.1), these children were invited for a thorough cardiometabolic assessment at our hospital. Systolic and diastolic blood pressure, blood lipid (low-density lipoprotein, high-density lipoprotein, triglycerides) and glucose (fasting glucose, fasting insulin, HbA1c) profiles, endothelial function of the microvasculature of the forearm, and cumulative cortisol and cortisone levels over the past 3 months assessed in hair were all similar between the two groups. Anthropometrics was, however, different. The children in the Vitrolife group had an increased weight when compared to the Cook group (adjusted weight difference = 1.58 kg, 95% CI 0.01–3.1). This was not due to a difference in height (adjusted height difference = -0.38 cm, 95% CI -2.38–1.62), but probably because of increased fat storage as waist circumference (adjusted difference 3.21cm, 95% CI 0.60–5.81) and truncal adiposity (adjusted difference 3.44mm, 95% CI 0.27–6.62) were higher in the Vitrolife group (Zandstra et al., 2018).

To the best of our knowledge, other publications on long-term health effects by culture media are not available, except for one publication by the group of Fauque et al. They started a randomized study, comparing Global medium (LifeGlobal) and Single Step Medium (SSM, Irvine Scientific), but this study ended prematurely because of the superiority of Global medium in terms of pregnancy rates. In the 73 live born singletons, no differences in birthweight, height, weight, head circumference, and medical history up to age 4 years, were found between the two culture media groups. This has to be taken with caution as the study was underpowered for many, if not all, of the health outcomes. Development, assessed in 55 children at 5 year of age, via the Child Development Inventory questionnaire which includes eight domains (social, self-help, gross motor, fine motor, expressive language, language comprehension, letter knowledge, number knowledge), was better in all domains in children from the Global group, even after correction for mother's socioeconomic status (Bouillon et al 2016). Although these results are obtained in a very limited number of children, it is remarkable that the direction of the effect of culture medium was the same in all domains (discussed in Roseboom, 2018). In our follow-up study of the 9-year old children from the Vitrolife-Cook study, no difference in school performance including language skills, mathematics and reading capability and comprehension was found between the two groups (Figure 11.1). Other development domains were not assessed.

11.3.2 Culture Time

Prolonged culture of embryos until the blastocyst stage is gaining ground. The potential advantage is the transfer of a blastocyst into the uterus which better mimics the in vivo situation with natural conception and the embryonic and endometrial phase being better synchronized on day 5. Extended culture is also assumed to allow a better selection of the embryo with the highest developmental potential. A meta-analysis showed increased live birth rates after fresh blastocyst transfer as compared to cleavage stage embryo transfer. However, there is no evidence for superiority in cumulative pregnancy rates when all transfers, fresh and frozen, from a single oocyte retrieval are included (Glujovsky et al., 2016; de Vos et al., 2016). Prolonged culture also exposes embryos to an artificial environment for two to three extra days, which raises concerns regarding the safety for the offspring. During the extra days, the activation of the embryonic genome might increase the sensitivity of an embryo to its environment.

A meta-analysis on perinatal outcomes after cleavage vs. blastocyst stage embryo transfer stratified for fresh and frozen embryo transfers showed that fresh blastocyst transfers have a higher risk for preterm birth <37 weeks (RR = 1.16, 95% CI 1.06–1.27), very preterm birth <32 weeks (RR = 1.16, 95%CI 1.02–1.31), and large for gestational age (RR = 1.22, 95%CI 1.00–1.48), when compared to fresh cleavage stage embryo transfers. The risk for small for gestational age was reduced (RR = 0.83, 95% CI 0.74–0.94). The risk for (very) low and high birth-weight is similar. When comparing frozen embryo transfers, only the risk for large for gestational age was increased after blastocyst transfer (Wang et al., 2017). Only one study reported mean birthweight, which was not affected by prolonged culture. The quality of the included studies is, however, variable. All studies are retrospective cohorts with high hetero-geneity. In some of the studies blastocyst transfer was only applied in good prognosis women and not all studies were able to correct for confounders.

Besides these perinatal outcomes, an increased risk for monozygotic twinning after blastocyst trans-fer has frequently been reported as well as an increased male-to-female ratio (Berntsen et al., 2019). Other offspring outcomes related to extended culture have to the best of our knowledge not been investigated and/or reported.

11.4 The Missing Link between Embryo Culture and Offspring Outcome

The fact that the embryo needs a specialized culture medium to survive but can develop within a range of different culture media, suggests that the embryo inter-acts with its environment and has a certain degree of developmental plasticity to cope with environmental alterations. Non-IVF animal studies have shown that environmental changes occurring during the few days around conception may lead to long-term health effects in the offspring. This confirms that the preimplantation embryo is sensitive to its environment, and that embry-onic adaptations might have long-lasting consequences for the offspring. The exact mechanism(s) linking these early adaptations to long-term effects have yet to be resolved. A process known to respond to environment and therefore a good candidate for the missing link is the epigenetic regulation (Roseboom, 2018).

The embryonic genome and epigenome are com-pletely remodeled during gamete formation and the first days of embryonic development. These remodel-ing processes – parental imprint establishment on the genome, global DNA demethylation and remethylation, maintenance of parent-of-origin spe-cific imprints, embryonic genome activation and the switch from maternal to embryonic transcripts, and cell differentiation towards the inner cell mass and trophectoderm – coincide with the time of IVF manipulations and are very adaptive to

environmental factors. Major epigenetic changes in DNA methylation, meaning hyper- or hypomethyla-tion of differentially methylated regions for instance, can lead to so-called imprinting disorders in the off-spring. Although the risk for one of these imprinting disorders is still very low, the number of cases with Beckwith-Wiedemann Syndrome or Angelman Syndrome who are conceived via IVF is higher than expected based on the percentage of IVF conceived children in the general population,. More mild epi-genetic alterations, not covering a whole methylated region or only a small fraction of cells, will not lead to congenital abnormalities, but may increase the sus-ceptibility for diseases in later life. These epigenetic alterations can be established directly in the embryo and passed on to daughter cells forming the new human being, or indirectly via epigenetic alterations in the placenta, that trigger adapting epigenetic responses in the fetus (Vrooman & Bartolomei, 2017).

In animal studies with mice and cattle, it has been extensively shown that embryo culture media and the supplementation with serum affect the epigenome of the embryo, with DNA methylation being most widely studied (summarized in [Mani & Mainigi, 2018]). Comparing mouse blastocysts developed in vitro in different culture media to those that developed in vivo showed perturbations in DNA methylation and imprinted, as well as global, gene expression (Mani & Mainigi, 2018). In adult off-spring, sex- and tissue-specific differences in gene expression profiles between mice resulting from in vitro culture and naturally conceived mice are found (Feuer & Rinaudo, 2017). Mouse embryos cultured under low oxygen in comparison to high oxygen, display global gene expression patterns and protein profiles that more closely resemble that of embryos developed in vivo (Wale & Gardner, 2016), specific-ally expression of enzymes involved in antioxidant metabolism (Salilew-Wondim et al., 2014). Changes are also found in the proteome and metabolism of embryos cultured in 5% and 20% oxygen respectively. Culture of embryos from an agouti mouse model, where causality between environmentally induced epigenetic effect and a phenotype can be shown, resulted in an increased hypomethylation of the A^{vy} allele, together with the corresponding alteration in coat color (Mani & Mainigi, 2018).

In human embryos, culture medium induced alterations in gene expression have been reported, as well as small DNA methylation alterations in placental and fetal tissue. However, as the affected regions differ between studies and between samples, it is likely that the epigenetic alterations occur stochastically. Furthermore, proving causality between culture-induced epigenetic alterations in the embryo and phenotypic outcomes in adult offspring is extremely difficult, if not impossible, considering the heterogeneity of the human population, not only in genetic background, but also in exposures during life (Mani & Mainigi, 2018).

11.5 Summary

It is clear from many studies using different animal species that in vitro culture affects embryonic epigenetic and gene expression profiles, and results in different perinatal and postnatal (including adult) phenotypes as compared to naturally conceived offspring. In humans, evidence is less easy to obtain, but reports indicate a possible impact of in vitro culture, and especially culture medium, on short- and long-term health outcomes. However, more research is needed to confirm these findings and to determine the implications for adult health. Nevertheless, it is important to create awareness among manufacturers and ART health care providers that embryo culture, as well as other ART manipulations, may affect offspring health. New techniques or for instance culture media should not be implemented unconditionally and follow-up studies of ART offspring are indispensable.

References

Adamson GD, Dyer S, Chambers et al. ICMART preliminary world report 2015. *Hum Repro.* 2019;34: i65.

Berntsen S, Soderstrom-Anttila V, Wennerholm UB, et al. The health of children conceived by ART: 'the chicken or the egg?' *Hum Reprod Update.* 2019;25:137–158.

Bouillon C, Léandri R, Desch L, et al. Does embryo culture medium influence the health and development of children born after in vitro fertilization? *PLoS ONE.* 2016;*11*:e0150857.

Calle A, Fernandez-Gonzalez R, Ramos-Ibeas P, et al. Long-term and transgenerational effects of in vitro culture on mouse embryos. *Theriogenology.* 2012;*77*:785–793.

De Vos A, Van Landuyt L, Santos-Ribeiro S, et al. Cumulative live birth rates after fresh and vitrified cleavage-stage versus blastocyst-stage embryo transfer in the first treatment cycle. *Hum Reprod.* 2016;31:2442–2449.

Dumoulin JC, Land JA, Van Montfoort AP, et al. Effect of in vitro culture of human embryos on birthweight of newborns. *Hum Reprod.* 2010;25:605–612.

Duranthon V, Chavatte-Palmer P. Long term effects of ART: What do animals tell us? *Mol Reprod Dev.* 2018;85:348–368.

Ealy AD, Wooldridge LK, McCoski SR. Board Invited Review: Post-transfer consequences of in vitro-produced embryos in cattle. *J Anim Sci.* 2019;97:2555–2568.

Feuer SK, Rinaudo PF. Physiological, metabolic and transcriptional postnatal phenotypes of in vitro fertilization (IVF) in the mouse. *J Dev Orig Health Dis.* 2017;8:403–410.

Gardner DK, Kelley RL. Impact of the IVF laboratory environment on human preimplantation embryo phenotype. *J Dev Orig Health Dis.* 2017;8:418–435.

Glujovsky D, Farquhar C, Quinteiro Retamar AM, Alvarez Sedo CR, Blake D. Cleavage stage versus blastocyst stage embryo transfer in assisted reproductive technology. *Cochrane Database Syst Rev.* 2016;CD002118.

Guo XY, Liu XM, Jin L, et al. Cardiovascular and metabolic profiles of offspring conceived by assisted reproductive technologies: a systematic review and meta-analysis. *Fertil Steril.* 2017;107: 22–631 e625.

Kleijkers SH, Mantikou E, Slappendel E., et al. Influence of embryo culture medium (G5 and HTF) on pregnancy and perinatal outcome after IVF: a multicenter RCT. *Hum Reprod.* 2016;31:2219–2230.

Mani S, Mainigi M. Embryo culture conditions and the epigenome. *Semin Reprod Med.* 2018;36:211–220.

Pinborg A, Wennerholm UB, Romundstad LB, et al. Why do singletons conceived after assisted reproduction technology have adverse perinatal outcome? Systematic review and meta-analysis. *Hum Reprod Update.* 2013;19:87–104.

Roseboom TJ. Developmental plasticity and its relevance to assisted human reproduction. *Hum Reprod.* 2018;33:546–552.

Salilew-Wondim D, Tesfaye D, Hoelker M, Schellander K. Embryo transcriptome response to environmental factors: implication for its survival under suboptimal conditions. *Anim Reprod Sci.* 2014;149:30–38.

Velazquez MA, Sheth B, Smith SJ, Eckert JJ, Osmond C, Fleming TP. Insulin and branched-chain amino acid depletion during mouse preimplantation embryo culture programmes body weight gain and raised blood pressure during early postnatal life.

Biochim Biophys Acta Mol Basis Dis. 2018;1864:590–600.

Vrooman LA, Bartolomei MS. Can assisted reproductive technologies cause adult-onset disease? Evidence from human and mouse. *Reprod Toxicol.* 2017;68:72–84.

Wale PL, Gardner DK. The effects of chemical and physical factors on mammalian embryo culture and their importance for the practice of assisted human reproduction. *Hum Reprod Update.* 2016;**22**:2–22.

Wang X, Du M, Guan Y, Wang B, Zhang J, Liu Z. Comparative neonatal outcomes in singleton births from blastocyst transfers or cleavage-stage embryo transfers: a systematic review and meta-analysis. *Reprod Biol Endocrinol.* 2017;15:36.

Wrenzycki C. Gene expression analysis and in vitro production procedures for bovine preimplantation embryos: Past highlights, present concepts and future prospects. *Reprod Domest Anim.* 2018;53 Suppl 2:14–19.

Zandstra H, Brentjens L, Spauwen B, et al. Association of culture medium with growth, weight and cardiovascular development of IVF children at the age of 9 years. *Hum Reprod.* 2018;33:1645–1656.

Zandstra H, Van Montfoort AP, Dumoulin JC. Does the type of culture medium used influence birthweight of children born after IVF? *Hum Reprod.* 2015;30:530–542.

Chapter 12

The Changing Culture of Embryo Culture
Advances in the IVF Culture System

Carol Lynn Curchoe and Jason E. Swain

12.1 Introduction

The IVF culture system is constantly being examined for means of modification to further improve conditions for gametes and embryos. Exhaustive research into physiological requirements and responses of these biological cells has provided valuable insight for refinement of culture variables. Extensive testing of conditions, both chemical and physical, has permitted tailoring of the IVF laboratory to the unique requirements of the reproductive cells as well as the needs and preferences of the IVF lab. Furthermore, as with many fields, improved efficiency and automation of normally manual processes within the laboratory is an active area of research. These various endeavors result in an ever changing landscape in the IVF laboratory.

While the culture system in the IVF laboratory entails >200 individual variables,[1,2] four broad classifications capture a majority of these items:

1) equipment
2) disposables
3) media
4) workflow/processes

These main categories have seen many changes since the early days of clinical IVF and are often intricately linked. With recent advances in technology and manufacturing, IVF equipment, and disposables in particular have experienced what can almost be classified as paradigm shifts in their configurations and use.

12.2 Equipment

12.2.1 Incubators

Amongst the changes within the confines of the IVF laboratory, one could argue that incubators have perhaps exhibited the greatest change. These laboratory workhorses have reduced in size considerably from large box-type units of ~150 L that were created to hold numerous flasks of adherent somatic cells to much smaller benchtop units optimized for embryo culture of one patient in each individual unit[3,4] (Figure 12.1). In addition to the dramatic size reduction, these IVF specific incubators are designed to reduce environmental stressors through:

- improved temperature recovery/stability
- proper gas mixture (low oxygen)
- gas/pH stability
- better air quality (internal filtration methods)
- and other relevant factors, such as cleaning and sterilization, monitoring and data logging capabilities, patient capacity.[4]

The advent of time-lapse imaging in conjunction with IVF-specific benchtop incubators has resulted in even more specialized and complex devices to potentially benefit IVF. These time-lapse incubators permit and promote the increased use of uninterrupted culture, where neither media nor embryo is disturbed via manual removal from the incubator for routine handling or observation. This uninterrupted approach attempts to further improve environmental stability and enhance outcomes, but impeccable quality control is paramount to avoid potential detrimental variables, such as evaporation, VOC accumulation and media degradation.[5] Validation of a superior culture environment and outcomes for these new incubators has not been verified in all studies,[4,6–9] but the increased data available from the imaging offers new opportunities to improve embryo selection using algorithms and artificial intelligence, or research into other novel visual indicators of embryo morphokinetics. It also creates a unique platform on which to build an even more customized system and workflow targeted to the unique needs and demands of the clinical IVF laboratory.

As an example of potential advancement, current time lapse imaging systems used in clinical IVF utilize basic brightfield or darkfield imaging to visualize cells

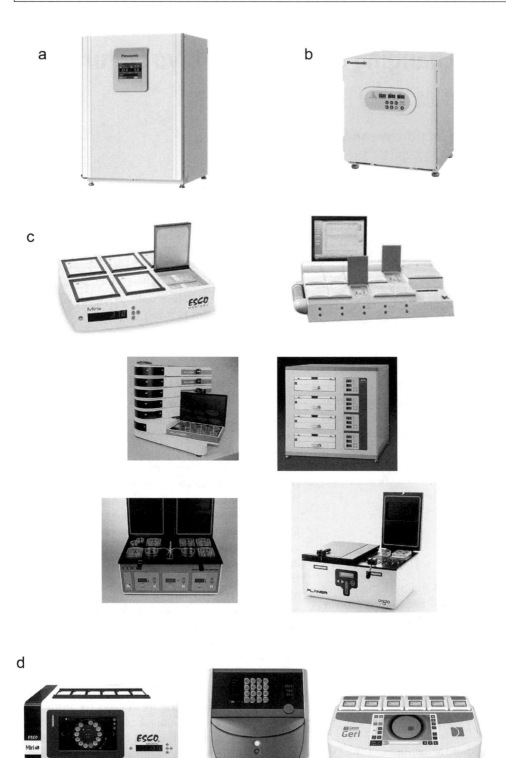

Figure 12.1 IVF culture incubators have evolved over time, reducing in size to units with individualized culture changes. **a.** Large box incubator, **b.** Small box incubator, **c.** various benchtop incubators, some with individualized chambers, **d.** time lapse incubators with individualized culture chambers. This evolution has results in improved growth conditions due, in part, to improved environmental stability. For color version of this figure. Please refer color plate section.

and track cell divisions. These are simple imaging technologies with limitations, such as low contrast, low resolution, and limits to magnification. However, more complex imaging approaches exist that could lend additional insight into cell quality, beyond cell division and basic morphology.[10,11] Several novel imaging approaches have been used to noninvasively examine gametes and embryos without negatively impacting function or development. Techniques like polarized light microscopy, RAMAN Fourier Transformed Infrared (FTIR), Coherent anti-RAMAN Stokes (CARS),[12] and combinations of these approaches can give information about oocyte spindle location and maturation status, cell lipid content, mitochondrial status, DNA damage, and other attributes.[10, 11] Features of these approaches are shown in Table 12.1. In research settings, these unique microscopy technologies have revolutionized the study of fine structures (down to the packing arrangement of DNA in sperm) in living cells. Whether these more complex imaging approaches could be miniaturized or made compatible with benchtop IVF incubators is unknown, but they offer an intriguing pathway to expand upon current time-lapse imaging approaches.

12.3 Consumables/Disposables

12.3.1 Novel Culture Platforms

While advancement in incubators has noticeably progressed, the physical platform on which gametes and embryos are cultured has remained largely unchanged. Since the start of culturing gametes and embryos in vitro, laboratories have utilized glass or plastic petri dishes, typically intended for adherent cell culture, and modified slightly for use with the reproductive cells. Recently, advancements in the physical platform on which embryos are cultured have begun to emerge.[13-17] Novel culture platform prototypes to benefit the unique requirements of oocytes and embryos have been made by 3D printing and other advanced manufacturing technologies. These embryo specific dishes have confined/constrictive designs to help create beneficial microenvironments, taking advantage of the benefits of group embryo culture and embryo spacing, while keeping cells separate for identification or selection purposes. [18, 19] These include microfunnels, channels, and other unique depressions to hold the cells (Figure 12.2). Several of these novel culture platforms are the direct result of the new IVF specific incubators

and go hand-in-hand with attempting to provide a superior culture environment based on the particular needs of delicate reproductive cells. At least one preliminary study indicates that a microvolume approach using the Well-of-a-Well (WOW) system may be superior for human embryo development compared to larger volume culture.[20] Currently, there is no consensus as to a superior culture dish or volume of media used for culture.

In addition to the dimensions of the culture device, exploration of novel materials or surface coatings may be useful in improving culture conditions. In vivo, the female reproductive tract provides a moist environment, where the embryo may encounter ciliated epithelium and various crypts and folds within the confines of the oviduct and then the intricate surface of the uterine lining, where various polyhydroxylated compounds, macromolecules, and components of the extracellular matrix are presented to the embryo. This is in stark contrast to the flat and inert surface of a plastic dish in the laboratory, where the embryo is submerged in a relative ocean of culture medium. In a field where the physiological basis has been a driving force in formulation of some culture media as well as the culture atmosphere, both resulting in improved embryo development, perhaps exploration of more physiological culture surfaces may also yield further improvements upon current practices.

Though limited, some research has examined the impact of altering culture surfaces and materials on preimplantation embryo development.[16] For example, surface coatings like Matrigel, hyaluronan, and agarose have been shown to impact embryo development. Mouse embryos cultured on Matrigel coated culture plates increased rates of mouse blastocyst hatching compared to those in media alone, though total rates of blastocyst formation were similar.[21] A later study using Matrigel yielded higher rates of blastocyst development and increased hatching rates.[22] However, subsequent studies examining the ability of Matrigel to support zygote development from random-bred mouse strains, which experience the 2-cell block, demonstrated an inhibitory effect of Matrigel on blastocyst development and hatching.[23] Though conflicting data exists, inclusion of hyaluronic acid in culture media has been shown to be beneficial for mouse and bovine embryo and fetal development,[24–26] and to improve pregnancy and implantation rates when included in human embryo transfer media.[27–31] Thus, the use of hyaluronan coated surfaces may be worthy of exploration.

Table 12.1 Various noninvasive imaging approaches used on gametes and embryos for potential use in conjunction with novel IVF incubators to be used as selection tools. (See review by Jasensky and Swain (2010)[10]

Imaging Approach	Information Obtained	Species
Polarized Light	- Oocyte spindle formation/location - Oocyte and embryo zona layers - Sperm acrosomal status - Sperm head vacuoles - Sperm DNA arrangement	Mouse Hamster Rat Bovine Human Insect
Multi-Photon	- Oocyte & embryo mitochondrial distribution - Embryo cell lineage	Rhesus Mouse
Harmonic Generation	- Spindle dynamics - Oocyte zona layers - Oocyte organelle localization - Embryo lipid droplet distribution	Mouse
Fourier Transformed Infrared (FTIR)	- Oocyte zona pellucida secondary protein structure - Oocyte lipid phase transition temperature	Human Bovine Porcine Murine
RAMAN	- Sperm mitochondrial status - Sperm DNA damage - Oocyte oxidative damage - Oocyte quality - Oocyte maturational status	Fish Human Mouse Xenopus Sheep
Coherent Anti-Raman Stokes (CARS)	- Oocyte lipid content	Mouse Bovine Porcine Human
Optical Quadrature Microscopy (OQM)	- Embryo cell counts	Mouse
Phase Subtraction (Optical Quadrature + DIC)	- Embryo cell boundaries/overlaps (cell/count)	Mouse
Optical Coherence Tomography (OCT)	- Clumping of unknown cytoplasmic structures following embryo vitrification	Mouse
Biodynamic Imaging (BDI)	- Cumulus cells, oocyte, zygote, and blastocyst observation of subcellular motion	Porcine
Quantitative Orientation Independent (DIC + Polarized microscopy)	- Spermatocyte microtubule and chromosome distribution	Crane fly
Multi-Modal (3-D fusion, DIC, epifluorescence, OQM, laser scanning confocal, two-photon)	- Imaging of blastocysts	Mouse

At least one preliminary abstract has examined the effects of coating the culture surface with a glycosaminoglycan matrix of hyaluronic acid. Though coating of flat polydimethylsiloxane (PDMS) surfaces and microwells with hyaluronic acid hydrogels was able to support mouse blastocyst formation at comparable levels to uncoated flat PDMS surfaces (81.4%,. 72.6%, and 86.3%, respectively), it significantly decreased blastocyst cell numbers compared to no coating.[32] Surface coatings using agarose have been used in supporting embryo development in vitro. Microwells made in agarose have been described for use in individual culture zona-free

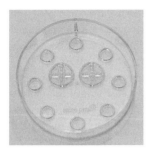
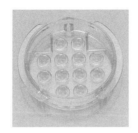
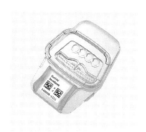
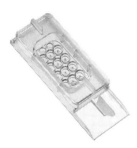
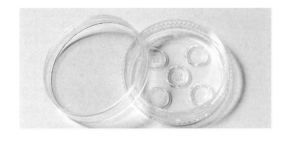

Figure 12.2 Various embryo specific culture dishes aimed at creating beneficial microenvironments and/or permitting individual cell separation/identification. Embryos are increasingly being cultured in specific dishes tested for use with embryos for toxicity and customized to create confined microfunnels or wells rather than using generic cell culture/petri dishes and larger volumes of media. For color version of this figure. Please refer color plate section.

embryos.[33] This method does allow for easy access to and identification of embryos, though no immediate benefit on growth over traditional culture surfaces has been noted. It should be noted that agarose gel tunnels were also used for extended culture of post hatching bovine embryos.[34] Interestingly, several types of agarose gel exist and it is unknown whether specific properties of these varying compounds can convey differential effects on embryo development.

Certain limitations exist with 2-dimentional culture, as contact with any specialized surface is minimal. In 3-dimensional culture approaches (Figure 12.3), growing cells are provided structural support and direct physical interaction with their surrounding environment, similar to that experienced in vivo. Additionally, 3-dimensional culture may allow for embedding and orientation of an array of glycoproteins or other macromolecules, compared to culture on a 2-dimensional surface. To date, most of the work with 3-dimensional culture has been performed with follicles or oocytes,[35–37] but similar approaches could be used with embryos, though modifications of the approach may be required to allow embryo visualization and grading, as well as embryo recovery for subsequent embryo transfer. Importantly, any surface coating or 3-dimensional approach must consider the impact of the matrix

on altering media composition and the resulting impact on gametes and embryos.

In addition to the surface environment differences experienced in vitro, the physical forces experienced by gametes and embryos in the laboratory also differ from what would be normally encountered in vivo. It is estimated that embryos in the female reproductive tract move and experience a sheer force of 0.1μm/s and 0–3 dyn/mm^2, respectively.[38,39] Thus, subtle or gentle movement could activate beneficial signaling pathways and perhaps benefit embryo development. This "Active Embryo Hypothesis" has some merit when considering the emerging literature.[13–17] On the other hand, embryos can experience excessive forces from procedures such as pipetting, which can impair development.[40, 41]

Various dynamic culture approaches exist, where cells are actively agitated or moved, rather than sitting in a relatively static state in a drop or well of media (Figure 12.4).

Dynamic embryo culture approaches used with human embryos include [14–16]:

- motorized tilting devices
- vibrating platforms
- methods to move media and cells though microfluidic devices using syringes or piezo-actuated pin systems.

A promising and widely trialed dynamic embryo culture approach appears to be subtle and periodic vibration. Initial studies in mouse, bovine, and human indicate that short bursts of vibration of around 5 seconds every ~60 min around 44Hz, improve embryo development and outcomes.[42–47] However, success rates of control samples were poor and a randomized clinical trial results demonstrated no improvement in usable blastocyst rate or sustained implantation rate between embryos cultured with a microvibration platform versus static culture.[48]

Notably, all of these dynamic culture systems require standard box-type (large or small) incubators for placement. With improved scaling and customization, these innovations may be applied in similar fashion to embryo specific benchtop incubators.

Microfluidic approaches lend themselves to combining several steps onto a single, novel platform to reduce handling and associated cell stress[15, 16] (Figure 12.5). Various procedures have been performed on microfluidic devices such as:

- oocyte maturation
- oocyte denuding
- cell orientation for ICSI or biopsy
- embryo culture
- vitrification.

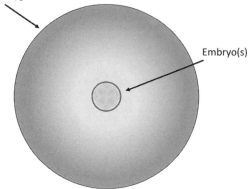

Biomimetic/gel-like Material

Embryo(s)

Figure 12.3 Three-dimensional culture approaches may offer a means of providing a more physiological approach to in vitro embryo culture by providing structural support and a more appropriate physical environment via different biomatrices. This method involves encapsulating cells into a bioscaffold or matrix material and has been used successfully for oocytes and follicles. Three-dimensional culture has not received widespread attention for use with embryos, but offers a means to provide structural support, a moist, rather than fluid environment, as well as present potentially beneficial molecules in an oriented fashion. However, 3-dimensional embryo culture does have unique considerations to address to facilitate embryo grading and recovery for subsequent uterine transfer or cryopreservation. For color version of this figure. Please refer color plate section.

12.4 Media

As discussed in Chapter 5, IVF culture media have seen refinement over the years from those used with somatic cells, to media used to culture early cleavage stage embryos, to more advanced systems that can successfully support development to the blastocyst stage. However, IVF culture media is still a target for future improvement as new culture technologies continue to develop.[49] For example, the increased use

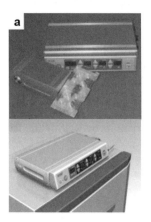
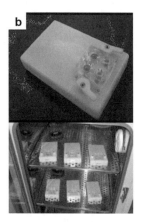
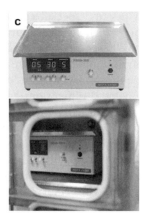

Figure 12.4 Representative images of dynamic embryo culture platforms that have been used clinically for human embryo culture. These platforms have historically required use of small or large box incubator and include **a.** tilting embryo culture, **b.** microfluidic culture and **c.** vibrational culture. Scaling down these approaches for use with smaller, modern benchtop incubators may provide an opportunity to improve upon current culture systems and facilitate more wide-spread implementation of this dynamic approach. For color version of this figure. Please refer color plate section.

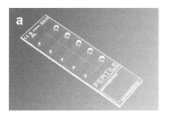
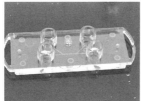
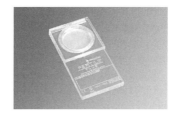
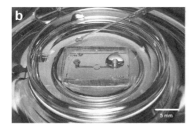
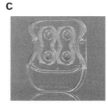

Figure 12.5 Various microfluidic platforms aimed at improving procedural steps involved in IVF have been examined, though most have not been widely implemented in clinical settings. **a.** Simple devices used for sperm sorting have received the most clinical use: semen is loaded into an inlet port and motile sperm collected from out an outlet port after traversing some arrangement of channels/obstacles to aid in sperm selection. While many experimental designs exist, at least two microfluidic systems have been tested on culturing human embryos: **b.** a simple static system and **c.** using actuated pins to drive fluid flow though microfluidic channels in a pulsatile fashion across embryos held in microfunnels. For color version of this figure. Please refer color plate section.

of time-lapse incubator technology and the associated uninterrupted culture, warrant investigation into improving the stability of culture media via inclusion of more stable compounds.[49, 50] Well-known issues with amino acid breakdown and ammonium production exist. Dipeptide forms of glutamine are now used to combat this. However, use of other dipeptides, like glycine, may be useful as well.[51.] Component stability is also a potential issue with pyruvate. Pyruvate is important for all embryo stages, especially early development; however, it is unstable and more stable forms may be advantageous for mammalian embryos.[52, 53] Novel combination buffering systems can be used to maintain pH stability.[54–57] Furthermore, media may come to be viewed as an independent treatment, with novel formulations based on a particular infertility etiology or other diagnostic assessment. Different embryos may benefit from different media formulations utilizing different antioxidant cocktails or specific growth factors.

12.5 Workflow/Processes

Various emerging technological advances can have a significant impact of laboratory workflow and processes. These are often aimed at improving upon current practices via optimizing efficiency of the system and or improving accuracy. Several examples

of how critical manual processes can be improved within the IVF laboratory are detailed below.

12.5.1 Electronic Witnessing

Double witnessing of key procedural steps in the IVF process is a requirement for an adequate quality control system. This is meant to avoid sample mix-ups and errors. However, manual witnessing is still subject to error. Electronic witnessing systems now exist for use in the IVF laboratory. Using RFID tags or printed barcodes or other image capture approaches, this necessary procedural step can be automated to create a more efficient and effective workflow. This technology is discussed in more detail in Chapter 7.

12.5.2 Digital Quality Control

It is widely accepted that laboratory quality control and assurance must be performed routinely, but appropriate levels of monitoring, what to monitor, and the best ways to monitor it are not clear. This has led to increasing demands on laboratory staff to monitor (sometimes multiple times a day), record, and ensure that the laboratory equipment and environment stays within preset operational parameters. Until recently, the dynamics/timing of the response of a liquid nitrogen dewar to physical tank failure was largely unknown (i.e., how a storage vessel behaves when the vacuum is breached) was unknown.[58] To address issues like this and others, digital and cloud-based solutions to discover malfunctioning instruments or environments are being adapted to ART from other industries where they are already best practice tools. In the prior example of dewar failure, new monitoring approaches not only include internal temperature, but external temperature measurement via probes or thermosensitive cameras and weight monitoring approaches that can all be monitored remotely. New cloud-based applications to collect, store, retrieve, and analyze instrument quality control data are available and lend support to standardization of quality control parameters and the opportunity to integrate with electronic health records to relate measured parameters to clinical outcomes.[59] Staff-based competency assessment is also in development to further digitalize staff-related competency assessments, training documentation, annual procedure evaluations, and real-time "in-cycle" embryologist statistics.

12.5.3 Artificial Intelligence

Artificial intelligence (AI), machine learning, and deep learning use big data to look for subtle outcomes or patterns that humans cannot detect. The applications for IVF range from automation of follicle counts, to gamete and embryo grading and selection, to determination of genetic status, quality control and embryologist KPIs, prediction of live birth, and even to donor: recipient gamete phenotype matching. With the increased adoption of imaging systems in IVF, application of AI to help analyze these images or perhaps more useful, videos, for key selection criteria may help improve quality of prediction and decrease time to clinical pregnancy. The achievement of a successful pregnancy is highly dependent on embryo quality. Numerous preliminary studies have emerged using AI for embryo image/video analysis as a possible selection tool and show great promise to predict which embryo can maximize the likelihood of a singleton pregnancy, for example, by age group. These studies have further demonstrated that AI systems do not require experts to annotate images (raw video can be used without human blastocyst assessment), that AI systems can reveal hidden significant details that human embryologists cannot evaluate, and that ploidy of an embryo can be predicted by AI.[60–67]

In addition to image analysis for embryo selection, AI can be used to look for other patterns in images and data to further improve laboratory operations.

12.5.4 Automation

Manual procedures predominate in the IVF laboratory. While this may be advantageous in certain aspects, consistency varies between technicians. Flexibility and openness to adopt to change is needed to further drive and develop radical improvements in IVF culture systems. Adoption of automation, as least in some of the more subjective, menial, or mundane aspects of the embryology laboratory can decrease inter- and intra-technician variability and strives to further address environmental stressors that can impair gamete function and embryo development.

The IVF laboratory has seen a more "automated" approach to embryo culture and morphology analysis via use of time lapse imaging systems and uninterrupted culture. This approach is meant to lessen environmental stressors imposed upon the embryo, and reduce the amount of time the embryologist must spend handling and assessing the cells. Unfortunately, traditional video analysis of time lapse images can also be time consuming and variable. This technology lends itself nicely to automated image analysis and selection. For example, the FDA-approved Eeva Test is driven by an Xtend algorithm (a standard multidimensional, static algorithm).[68] Eeva uses time-lapse imaging (videos of embryo development) with the aim to predict which embryo has the best chance of progressing to a blastocyst.

Some of the aforementioned dynamic culture platforms implement multiple procedural steps on a single platform, with the intent to reduce manual cell handling and associated environmental stressors. Some simple devices have been utilized to keep delicate cells in place, while gradually changing media, or gently rolling the cell to a new location to produce a less stressful environment and help optimize growth conditions.[69, 70] More recently, mouse embryos have been successfully fertilized and cultured on a single platform without removing cells between the procedural steps.[71–73] Several examples of microfluidic platforms aimed at automating more complex procedures, demonstrate that visual tracking of a single sperm, robotic immobilization of sperm, aspiration of sperm with picoliter volume, and insertion of sperm into an oocyte (robotic ICSI) with a high degree of reproducibility are possible.[74–79] Additionally, automated devices have been designed to flow cryoprotectant over cells in a gradual manner, reducing osmotic shock, and offering a potential improvement of manual step-wise approach to dehydrating gametes and embryos for vitrification.[80–82] Utilizing this approach with existing semi-automated vitrification systems[83] may offer the opportunity to further improve success rates.

More ambitious and complex culture devices are emerging. Recently, a miniaturized array has been developed that can hold multiple zebrafish embryos in individual locations while utilizing microfluidic perfusion to supply fresh media or pharmacologic compounds to examine effects over time.[84] This array integrates a perfusion pump, stage heater, and valves to help regulate media flow and remove waste, and is also combined with real-time video analysis. A similar approach could be envisioned for mammalian embryo culture. Already, the field of IVF has adopted uninterrupted culture systems that leave embryos in a single culture medium on a single dish for 5–6 days in an attempt to reduce handling and stress. The rapid adaption of time-lapse imaging in IVF specific incubators coupled with novel culture platforms represents a potential platform to facilitate automation. Automation of image analysis on at least two clinical time-lapse systems is already a reality.[85–88]

12.6 Conclusion

Some of the IVF laboratory approaches discussed in this chapter may never reach clinical application, but the need to keep searching and striving for improvement and to facilitate change in the IVF laboratory is paramount if we hope to continue to improve outcomes. One can envision a culture system that combines various aspects using benchtop incubator technology that incorporates dynamic culture with embryo-specific dishes, employing advanced imaging and other non-invasive sampling approaches. Such a system would likely require AI at its core to ensure proper interpretation of this wealth of data. On a cutting edge incubator, perhaps an AI system could even adjust culture system variables like pH or temperature in real time to correct environmental anomalies. Importantly, embryologists will need to continue to improve and expand their training and skills to be tech savvy for routine equipment QC and troubleshooting and always remain vigilant in observing and looking for variation, as systems can fail.

References

1. Pool TB, Schoolfield J, Han D. Human embryo culture media comparisons. *Methods Mol Biol.* 2012;912:367–386.

2. Rieger D. Culture systems: physiological and environmental factors that can affect the outcome of human ART. *Methods Mol Biol.* 2012;912:333–354.

3. Swain J, Lagunov A. IVF incubator handling. In: Rizk B, Montag M, eds. *Standard Operational Procedures in Reproductive Medicine Laboratory and Clinical Practice.* Boca Raton: CRC Press; 2017: 8–11.

4. Swain JE. Decisions for the IVF laboratory: comparative analysis of embryo culture incubators. *Reprod Biomed Online.* 2014;28:535–547.

5. Swain JE. Controversies in ART: considerations and risks for uninterrupted embryo culture. *Reprod Biomed Online.* 2019;39:19–26.

6. Cruz M, Gadea B, Garrido N, et al. Embryo quality, blastocyst and ongoing pregnancy rates in oocyte donation patients whose embryos were monitored by time-lapse imaging. *J Assist Reprod Genet.* 2011;28:569–573.

7. Kirkegaard K, Hindkjaer JJ, Grondahl ML, Kesmodel US, Ingerslev HJ. A randomized clinical trial comparing embryo culture in a conventional incubator with a time-lapse incubator. *J Assist Reprod Genet.* 2012;29:565–572.

8. Park H, Bergh C, Selleskog U, Thurin-Kjellberg A, Lundin K. No benefit of culturing embryos in a closed system compared with a conventional incubator in terms of number of good quality embryos: results from an RCT. *Hum Reprod.* 2015;30:268–275.

9. Wu L, Han W, Wang J, et al. Embryo culture using a time-lapse monitoring system improves live birth rates compared with a conventional culture system: a prospective cohort study. *Hum Fertil.* 2018;21:255–262.

10. Jasensky J, Swain JE. Peering beneath the surface: novel imaging techniques to noninvasively select gametes and embryos for ART. *Biol Reprod.* 2013;89:105.

11. Swain JE. Novel imaging techniques to assess gametes and preimplantation embryos. In: Schatten, H, ed. *Human Reproduction: Updates and New Horizons.* Hobken, NJ:Wiley Blackwell; 2017: 231–256.

12. Jasensky J, Boughton AP, Khmaladze A, et al. Live-cell quantification and comparison of mammalian oocyte cytosolic lipid content between species, during development, and in relation to body composition using nonlinear vibrational microscopy. *Analyst*. 2016;141:4694–4706.

13. Swain JE. Shake, rattle and roll: bringing a little rock to the IVF laboratory to improve embryo development. *J Assist Reprod Genet*. 2014;31:21–24.

14. Swain JE, Lai D, Takayama S, Smith GD. Thinking big by thinking small: application of microfluidic technology to improve ART. *Lab Chip*. 2013;13:1213–1224.

15. Smith GD, Takayama S, Swain JE. Rethinking in vitro embryo culture: new developments in culture platforms and potential to improve assisted reproductive technologies. *Biol Reprod*. 2012;86:62.

16. Swain JE, Smith GD. Advances in embryo culture platforms: novel approaches to improve preimplantation embryo development through modifications of the microenvironment. *Hum Reprod Update*. 2011;17:541–557.

17. Smith GD, Swain JE, Bormann CL. Microfluidics for gametes, embryos, and embryonic stem cells. *Semin Reprod Med*. 2011;29:5–14.

18. Ebner T, Shebl O, Moser M, Mayer RB, Arzt W, Tews G. Group culture of human zygotes is superior to individual culture in terms of blastulation, implantation and life birth. *Reprod Biomed Online*. 2010;21:762–768.

19. Reed M, Woodward B, Swain J. Single or group culture of mammalian embryos: the verdict of the literature. *J Reprod Biotech Fertil*. 2011;2:77–87.

20. Vajta G, Korosi T, Du Y, et al. The Well-of-the-Well system: an efficient approach to improve embryo development. *Reprod Biomed Online*. 2008;17:73–81.

21. Carnegie J, Claman P, Lawrence C, Cabaca O. Can Matrigel substitute for Vero cells in promoting the in-vitro development of mouse embryos? *Hum Reprod*. 1995;10:636–641.

22. Lazzaroni L, Fusi FM, Doldi N, Ferrari A. The use of Matrigel at low concentration enhances in vitro blastocyst formation and hatching in a mouse embryo model. *Fertil Steril*. 1999;71:1133–1137.

23. Dawson KM, Baltz JM, Claman P. Culture with Matrigel inhibits development of mouse zygotes. *J Assist Reprod Genet*. 1997;14:543–548.

24. Lane M, Maybach JM, Hooper K, Hasler JF, Gardner DK. Cryo-survival and development of bovine blastocysts are enhanced by culture with recombinant albumin and hyaluronan. *Mol Reprod Dev*. 2003;64:70–78.

25. Gardner DK, Rodriegez-Martinez H, Lane M. Fetal development after transfer is increased by replacing protein with the glycosaminoglycan hyaluronan for mouse embryo culture and transfer. *Hum Reprod*. 1999;14:2575–2580.

26. Palasz AT, Rodriguez-Martinez H, Beltran-Brena P, et al. Effects of hyaluronan, BSA, and serum on bovine embryo in vitro development, ultrastructure, and gene expression patterns. *Mol Reprod Dev*. 2006;73:1503–1511.

27. Hambiliki F, Ljunger E, Karlstrom PO, Stavreus-Evers A. Hyaluronan-enriched transfer medium in cleavage-stage frozen-thawed embryo transfers increases implantation rate without improvement of delivery rate. *Fertil Steril*. 2010;94:1669–1673.

28. Sifer C, Mour P, Tranchant S, et al. Is there an interest in the addition of hyaluronan to human embryo culture in IVF/ICSI attempts? [In French]. *Gynecol Obstet Fertil*. 2009;37:884–889.

29. Korosec S, Virant-Klun I, Tomazevic T, Zech NH, Meden-Vrtovec H. Single fresh and frozen-thawed blastocyst transfer using hyaluronan-rich transfer medium. *Reprod Biomed Online*. 2007;15:701–707.

30. Loutradi KE, Prassas I, Bili E, Sanopoulou T, Bontis I, Tarlatzis BC. Evaluation of a transfer medium containing high concentration of hyaluronan in human in vitro fertilization. *Fertil Steril*. 2007;87:8–52.

31. Bontekoe S, Heineman MJ, Johnson N, Blake D. Adherence compounds in embryo transfer media for assisted reproductive technologies. *Cochrane Database Syst Rev*. 2014;2:Cd007421.

32. Oakes M, Cabrera L, Nanadivada H, Lahann J, Smith G. Effects of 3-dimensional topography, dynamic fluid movement and an insoluble glycoprotein matrix on murine embyro development. *Proceedings from the SGI Annual Meeting*, Glasgow, Scotland. 2009.

33. Peura TT, Vajta G. A comparison of established and new approaches in ovine and bovine nuclear transfer. *Cloning Stem Cells*. 2003;5:257–277.

34. Brandao DO, Maddox-Hyttel P, Lovendahl P, Rumpf R, Stringfellow D, Callesen H. Post hatching development: a novel system for extended in vitro culture of bovine embryos. *Biol Reprod*. 2004;71:2048–2055.

35. Laronda MM, Rutz AL, Xiao S, et al. A bioprosthetic ovary created using 3D printed microporous scaffolds restores ovarian function in sterilized mice. *Nat Commun*. 2017;8:15261.

36. Brito IR, Lima IM, Xu M, Shea LD, Woodruff TK, Figueiredo JR. Three-dimensional systems for in vitro follicular culture: overview of alginate-based matrices. *Reprod Fertil Dev*. 2014;26:915–930.

37. Shikanov A, Xu M, Woodruff TK, Shea LD. A method for ovarian follicle encapsulation and culture in a proteolytically degradable 3 dimensional system. *J Vis Exp.* 2011;15:2695

38. Greenwald GS A study of the transport of ova through the rabbit oviduct. *Fertil Steril.* 1961;12:80–95.

39. Matsuura K, Hayashi N, Kuroda Y, et al. Improved development of mouse and human embryos using a tilting embryo culture system. *Reprod Biomed Online.* 2010;20:358–364.

40. Xie Y, Wang F, Zhong W, Puscheck E, Shen H, Rappolee DA. Shear stress induces preimplantation embryo death that is delayed by the zona pellucida and associated with stress-activated protein kinase-mediated apoptosis. *Biol Reprod.* 2006;75:45–55.

41. Xie Y, Wang F, Puscheck EE, Rappolee DA. Pipetting causes shear stress and elevation of phosphorylated stress-activated protein kinase/jun kinase in preimplantation embryos. *Mol Reprod Dev.* 2007;74:1287–1294.

42. Isachenko E, Maettner R, Isachenko V, Roth S, Kreienberg R, Sterzik K. Mechanical agitation during the in vitro culture of human pre-implantation embryos drastically increases the pregnancy rate. *Clin Lab.* 2010;56:569–576.

43. Isachenko, V, Maettner R, Sterzik K, et al. In-vitro culture of human embryos with mechanical micro-vibration increases implantation rates. *Reprod BioMed Online.* 2011;22:536–544.

44. Hur YS, Park JH, Ryu EK, et al. Effect of micro-vibration culture system on embryo development. *J Assist Reprod Genet.* 2013;30:835–841.

45. Isachenko V, Sterzik K, Maettner R, et al. In vitro microvibration increases implantation rate after embryonic cell transplantation. *Cell Transplant.* 2017;26:789–794.

46. Hur YS, Ryu EK, Yoon SH, Lim KS, Lee WD, Lim JH. Comparison of static culture, micro-vibration culture, and micro-vibration culture with co-culture in poor ovarian responders. *Clin Exp Reprod Med.* 2016;43:146–151.

47. Takahashi M, Honda T, Hatoya S, Inaba T, Kawate N, Tamada H. Efficacy of mechanical micro-vibration in the development of bovine embryos during in vitro maturation and culture. *J Vet Med Sci.* 2018;80:532–535.

48. Juneau CR, Franasiak JM, Morin SJ, Werner MD, Upham KM, Scott RT. EnMotion: Embryos natural motion. blastulation is not different between static and dynamic cutlure systems. *Fertil Steril.* 2016;106:e358–359.

49. Swain JE Optimal human embryo culture. *Semin Reprod Med.* 2015;33:103–117.

50. Swain JE Controversies in ART: considerations and risks for uninterrupted embryo culture. *Reprod Biomed Online.* 2019;39:18–26.

51. Moravek M, Fisseha S, Swain JE. Dipeptide forms of glycine support mouse preimplantation embryo development in vitro and provide protection against high media osmolality. *J Assist Reprod Genet.* 2012;29:283–290.

52. Swain J, Pool T. Supplementation of culture media with esterified forms of pyruvate improves mouse embryo development. *Fertil Steril.* 2008;90 (Suppl):S47.

53. Silva E, Becker J, Herrick J, et al. Replacement of sodium pyruvate with ethyl pyruvate promotes zygotic cleavage and inner cell mass development during in vitro culture of embryos from females of advanced maternal age. *Fertil Steril.* 2016;106: e361.

54. Swain, JE Optimizing the culture environment in the IVF laboratory: impact of pH and buffer capacity on gamete and embryo quality. *Reprod Biomed Online.* 2010;21:6–16.

55. Swain JE, Pool TB. Supplementation of culture media with zwitterionic buffers supports sperm function and embryo development within the elevated CO_2 levels of the laboratory incubator. *J Clin Embryol.* 2008;11:24–26.

56. Swain JE, Pool TB. New pH-buffering system for media utilized during gamete and embryo manipulations for assisted reproduction. *Reprod Biomed Online.* 2009;18:799–810.

57. Will, MA, Clark NA, JE Swain. Biological pH buffers in IVF: help or hindrance to success. *J Assist Reprod Genet.* 2011;28:711–724.

58. Pomeroy KO, Reed ML, LoManto B, Harris SG, Hazelrigg WB, Kelk DA. Cryostorage tank failures: temperature and volume loss over time after induced failure by removal of insulative vacuum. *J Assist Reprod Genet.* 2019;36:2271–2278.

59. Palmer GA, Kratka C, Szvetecz S, et al. Comparison of 36 assisted reproduction laboratories monitoring environmental conditions and instrument parameters using the same quality-control application. *Reprod Biomed Online.* 2019;39:63–74.

60. Khosravi P, Kazemi E, Zhan Q, et al. Deep learning enables robust assessment and selection of human blastocysts after in vitro fertilization. *NPJ Digit Med.* 2019;2:21.

61. Tran D, Cooke S, Illingworth PJ, Gardner DK. Deep learning as a predictive tool for fetal heart pregnancy following time-lapse incubation and blastocyst transfer. *Hum Reprod.* 2019;34:1011–1018.

62. Miyagi Y, Habara T, Hirata R, Hayashi N. Feasibility of artificial intelligence for predicting live birth without aneuploidy from a blastocyst image. *Reprod Med Biol.* 2019;18:204–211.

63. Miyagi Y, Habara T, Hirata R, Hayashi N. Feasibility of deep learning for predicting live birth from a blastocyst image in patients classified by age. *Reprod Med Biol.* 2019;18:190–203.

64. Simopoulou M, Sfakianoudis K, Maziotis E, et al. Are computational applications the "crystal ball" in the IVF laboratory? The evolution from mathematics to artificial intelligence. *J Assist Reprod Genet.* 2018;35:1545–1557.

65. Manna C, Nanni L, Lumini A, Pappalardo S. Artificial intelligence techniques for embryo and oocyte classification. *Reprod Biomed Online.* 2013;26:42–49.

66. Curchoe CL, Bormann CL. Artificial intelligence and machine learning for human reproduction and embryology presented at ASRM and ESHRE 2018. *J Assist Reprod Genet.* 2019;36:591–600.

67. Kanakasabapathy MK, Thirumalaraju P, Bormann CL, et al. Development and evaluation of inexpensive automated deep learning-based imaging systems for embryology. *Lab Chip.* 2019;19:4139–4145.

68. Diamond MP, Suraj V, Behnke EJ, et al. Using the Eeva Test adjunctly to traditional day 3 morphology is informative for consistent embryo assessment within a panel of embryologists with diverse experience. *J Assist Reprod Genet.* 2015;32:61–68.

69. Clark S, Walters E, Beebe D, Wheeler M. A novel integrated in vitro maturation and in vitro fertilization system for swine. *Theriogenology.* 2003;59:441.

70. Sano H, Matsuura K, Naruse K, Funahashi H. Application of a microfluidic sperm sorter to the in-vitro fertilization of porcine oocytes reduced the incidence of polyspermic penetration. *Theriogenology.* 2010;74:863–870.

71. Han C, Zhang Q, Ma R, et al. Integration of single oocyte trapping, in vitro fertilization and embryo culture in a microwell-structured microfluidic device. *Lab Chip.* 2010;10:2848–2854.

72. Ma R, Xie L, Han C, et al. In vitro fertilization on a single-oocyte positioning system integrated with motile sperm selection and early embryo development. *Anal Chem.* 2011;83:964–970.

73. Mizuno J, Ostrovidov S, Nakamura H, et al. Human ART on chip: development of microfluidic device for IVF and IVC. *Proceedings from ESHRE.* 2007.

74. Lu Z, Zhang X, Leung C, Esfandiari N, Casper RF, Sun Y. Robotic ICSI (intracytoplasmic sperm injection). *IEEE Trans Biomed Eng.* 2011;58:2102–2108.

75. Mattos LS, Grant E, Thresher R, Kluckman K. Blastocyst microinjection automation. *IEEE Trans Inf Technol Biomed.* 2009;13:822–831.

76. Liu X, Fernandes R, Gertsenstein M, et al. Automated microinjection of recombinant BCL-X into mouse zygotes enhances embryo development. *PLoS ONE.* 2011;6:e21687.

77. Leung C, Lu Z, Esfandiari N, Casper RF, Sun Y. Automated sperm immobilization for intracytoplasmic sperm injection. *IEEE Trans Biomed Eng.* 2011;58:935–942.

78. Graf SF, Madigou T, Li R, Chesne C, Stemmer A, Knapp HF. Fully automated microinjection system for *Xenopus laevis* oocytes with integrated sorting and collection. *J Lab Autom.* 2011;16:186–196.

79. Park J, Jung SH, Kim YH, Kim B, Lee SK, Park JO. Design and fabrication of an integrated cell processor for single embryo cell manipulation. *Lab Chip.* 2005;5:91–96.

80. Lai D, Ding J, Smith GW, Smith GD, Takayama S. Slow and steady cell shrinkage reduces osmotic stress in bovine and murine oocyte and zygote vitrification. *Hum Reprod.* 2015;30:37–45.

81. Heo YS, Lee HJ, Hassell BA, et al. Controlled loading of cryoprotectants (CPAs) to oocyte with linear and complex CPA profiles on a microfluidic platform. *Lab Chip.* 2011;11:3530–3537.

82. Meng L, Huezo X, Stone B, Back K, Ringler G, Marrs R. Development of a microfluidic device for automated vitrficatio nof human embryros. *Fertil Steril.* 2011;96:s207.

83. Roy TK, Brandi S, Tappe NM, et al. Embryo vitrification using a novel semi-automated closed system yields in vitro outcomes equivalent to the manual Cryotop method. *Hum Reprod.* 2014;29:2431–2438.

84. Akagi, J, Khoshmanesh K, Evans B, et al. Miniaturized embryo array for automated trapping, immobilization and microperfusion of zebrafish embryos. *PLoS One.* 2012;7: e36630.

85. Wong CC, Loewke KE, Bossert NL, et al. Non-invasive imaging of human embryos before embryonic genome activation predicts development to the blastocyst stage. *Nat Biotechnol.* 2010;28:1115–1121.

86. Chavez SL, Loewke KE, Han J, et al. Dynamic blastomere behaviour reflects human embryo ploidy by the four-cell stage. *Nat Commun.* 2012;3:1251.

87. Paternot G, Debrock S, De Neubourg D, D'Hooghe TM, Spiessens C. Semi-automated morphometric analysis of human embryos can reveal correlations between total embryo volume and clinical pregnancy. *Hum Reprod.* 2013;28:627–633.

88. Wong C, Chen AA, Behr B, Shen S. Time-lapse microscopy and image analysis in basic and clinical embryo development research. *Reprod Biomed Online.* 2013;26:120–129.

Index